CURRENT GENETICS IN DERMATOLOGY

Edited by **Naoki Oiso**

Current Genetics in Dermatology
http://dx.doi.org/10.5772/3340
Edited by Naoki Oiso

Contributors
Yutaka Shimomura, Ken Natsuga, Daisuke Tsuruta, Chiharu Tateishi, Masamitsu Ishii, Tamihiro Kawakami, Naoki Oiso, Akira Kawada, Tomoki Kosho, Akira Kawada, Shigeru Kawara, Hajime Nakano, Michihiro Kono, Masashi Akiyama, Masaaki Kawase, Miki Tanioka, Teruhiko Makino, Takahiro Kurimoto, Muneharu Miyake, Akira Kawada

Published by InTech
Janeza Trdine 9, 51000 Rijeka, Croatia

Publishing Process Manager Iva Lipovic
Typesetting InTech DTP Team
Cover InTech Design Team

Additional hard copies can be obtained from orders@intechopen.com

Current Genetics in Dermatology, Edited by Naoki Oiso
p. cm.
ISBN 978-953-51-0971-6

For EU product safety concerns:
IN TECH d.o.o., Prolaz Marije Krucifikse Kozulić 3, 51000 Rijeka, Croatia,
info@intechopen.com or visit our website at intechopen.com.

Meet the editor

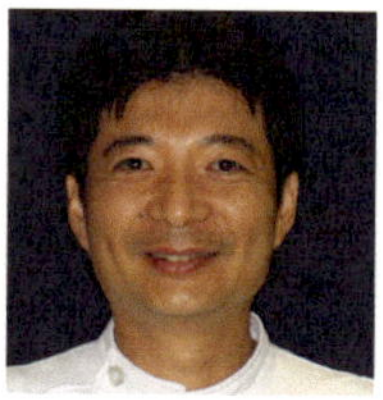

Naoki Oiso was born on 31 May, 1968 in Toyooka, Hyogo, Japan. He received M.D. and Ph.D. degree. In 2012, Oiso serves as an Associate Professor at Departments of Dermatology and Patient Safety & Management, Kinki University Faculty of Medicine, in Osaka-Sayama, Osaka, Japan. In 1988, he was a student at Osaka City University School of Medicine in Osaka, Japan. In 1997, Dr. Oiso was a graduate student at Osaka City University Graduate School of Medicine in Osaka, Japan. In 2001, he was a Postdoctoral Fellow at Human Medical Genetics Program, University of Colorado Health Sciences Center in Denver, USA. In 2005, Oiso served as an Assistant Professor at Department of Dermatology, Kinki University Faculty of Medicine, in Osaka-Sayama, Osaka, Japan.

Contents

Preface

Recent genetic progress in the dermatologic field provides many novel findings. "Current Genetics in Dermatology" is designed to summarize findings in each genodermatosis. All of chapters are described by young and energetic dermatologists who are specialists in each field.

We have to thank Ms. Iva Lipovic, Mr. Oliver Kurelic, Mrs. Ana Skalamera, and Ms. Petra Nenadic for excellent help throughout the processes for publication. We also appreciate all authors for sharing time for this book.

We hope you enjoy reading "Current Genetics in Dermatology".

Naoki Oiso, M.D., Ph.D.
Associate Professor

Akira Kawada, M.D., Ph.D.
Chief Professor

Department of Dermatology
Kinki University Faculty of Medicine
Osaka-Sayama, Osaka,
Japan

Chapter 1

Current Genetics in Hair Diseases

Yutaka Shimomura

Additional information is available at the end of the chapter

http://dx.doi.org/10.5772/54004

1. Introduction

(HF) is a skin appendage which exists on the entire skin surface, except for palmoplantar and mucosal regions. During embryogenesis, HF development is operated through reciprocal interactions between skin epithelial cells and underlying dermal cells [1]. The first signal to induce HF formation is considered to originate from the dermal cells. The epithelial cells which receive the dermal signal lead to form a placode (Figure 1). Then a signal from the placode results in forming a dermal condensate just beneath the placode (Figure 1). Additional interaction between these structures induces the downgrowth of the placode and forms a hair germ, which is the source of epithelial components of the HF (Figure 2). The dermal condensate is gradually surrounded by the HF epithelium and becomes a dermal papilla. It has been shown that many signaling molecules, such as Wnt, ectodysplasin (Eda),

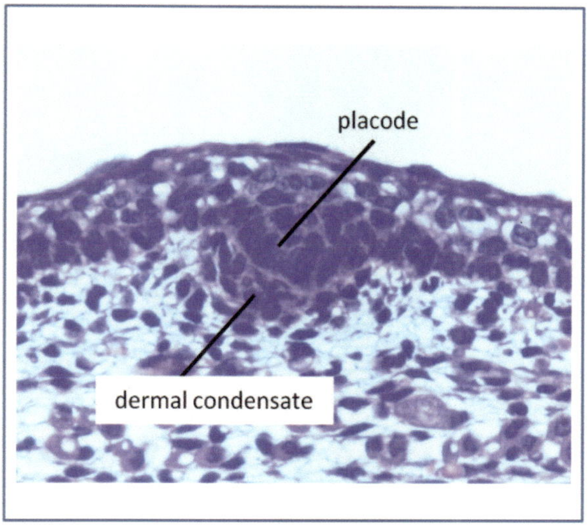

Figure 1. Hair follicle placode (mouse embryo; E15.5)

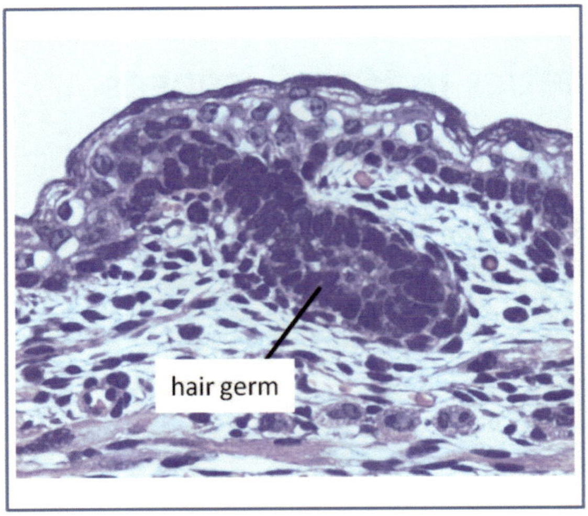

Figure 2. Hair germ (mouse embryo; E16.5)

bone morphogenic protein (Bmp), and sonic hedgehog (Shh), play crucial roles in the HF development [1]. After the HF is generated, it undergoes dynamic cell kinetics, known as the hair cycle, throughout postnatal life, which is composed of three phases: catagen (regressing) phase, telogen (resting) phase and anagen (growing) phase [2]. In human scalp HFs, duration of the catagen, telogen, and anagen phases are 1-2 weeks, 2-3 months, and 2-6 years, respectively. The hair cycle, which is an amazing ability of self-renewal, is maintained by the stem cell niche in bulge portion of the HF, as well as the dermal papilla [3, 4].

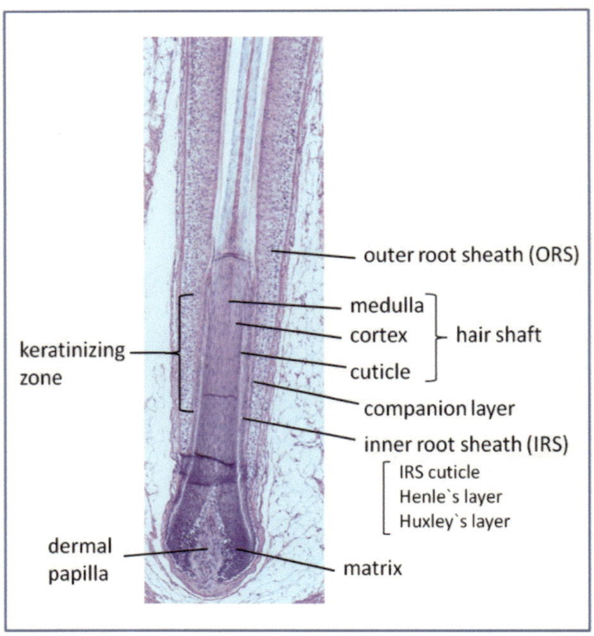

Figure 3. Human anagen hair follicle.

The anagen HF has a highly complex structure with several distinct cell layers (Figure 3). During the anagen phase, cells from the bulge portion migrate downward to matrix region, while making the outer root sheath (ORS). The matrix cells actively proliferate and differentiate into the hair shaft, the inner root sheath (IRS), and the companion layer of the HF (Figure 3) [4]. The hair shaft shares a common structural organization, in which a multicellular cortex is surrounded by a cuticular layer, occasionally with a medulla layer centrally located within the cortex. The hair shaft is strongly keratinized at the level of keratinizing zone, and forms a rigid structure (Figure 3). Growth of the hair shaft is molded and supported by the IRS, the companion layer, and the ORS. The IRS is composed of three distinct layers: the IRS cuticle, Huxley's layer, and Henle's layer (Figure 3).

2. Hair follicle

Recent advances in molecular genetics have led to the identification of numerous genes that are expressed in the HF. Furthermore, mutations in some of these genes have been shown to underlie hereditary hair diseases in humans [2]. Causative genes for the diseases encode various proteins with different functions, such as structural proteins, transcription factors, and signaling molecules. This chapter aims to update recent findings regarding the molecular basis of genetic hair diseases.

3. Keratin disorders

Keratins are one of the major structural components of the HF, and are largely divided into type I (acidic) and type II (neutral to basic) keratins. The type I and type II keratins undergo heterodimerization, which leads to form keratin intermediate filaments (KIFs) in the cytoplasm [5]. Based on the amino acid composition, keratins are further classified into two groups: epithelial (soft) keratins and hair (hard) keratins. As compared to the epithelial keratins, the hair keratins show higher sulfur content in their N- and C-terminus, which plays an important role in interacting with hair keratin-associated proteins via disulfide bindings [6, 7]. All the keratin proteins are composed of an N-terminal rod domain, a central rod domain, and a C-terminal tail domain. Importantly, the N-terminal and the C-terminal regions of the rod domain are highly conserved in amino acid sequences, which are called helix initiation motif (HIM) and helix termination motif (HTM), respectively (Figure 4). It is believed that the HIM and the HTM play essential roles in heterodimerization between the keratins. In humans, gene clusters for the type I and type II keratin genes are mapped on chromosomes 17q21 [8] and 12q13 [9], respectively. To date, a total of 54 functional keratin genes (28 type I and 26 type II) have been identified and characterized in humans. It has been shown that during differentiation of the HF, various keratin genes are abundantly and differentially expressed, and contribute to HF keratinization, leading to the formation of a rigid structure [10]. In general, epithelial keratins are mainly expressed in the ORS, the companion layer, the IRS, while hair keratins are predominantly expressed in the hair shaft. In addition, it has recently been reported that some epithelial keratins are expressed in the hair shaft medulla as well [11]. It is noteworthy that mutations in several keratin genes have been reported to underlie hereditary hair disorders in humans (Table 1).

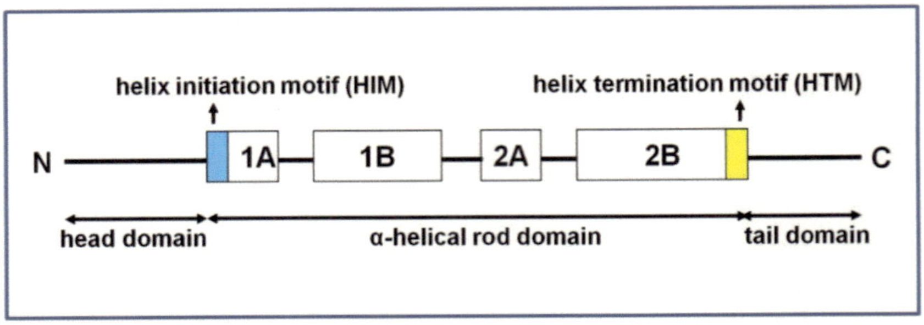

Figure 4. Structure of keratin proteins.

disease	inheritance pattern	OMIM#	main symptoms	gene	protein, function
Monilethrix	AD	158000	moniliform hair, perifollicular papules	*KRT81* *KRT83* *KRT86*	K81 (basic hair keratin) K83 (basic hair keratin) K86 (basic hair keratin)
Pure hair and nail ectodermal dysplasia	AR	602032	hypotrichosis, spoon nails	*KRT85*	K85 (basic hair keratin)
Autosomal dominant woolly hair (ADWH)/ hypotrichosis	AD	194300/613981	WH/ hypotrichosis	*KRT74* *KRT71*	K74 (basic epithelial keratin) K71 (basic epithelial keratin)

Table 1. Hereditary hair disorders caused by mutations in keratin genes. AD, autosomal dominant; AR, autosomal recessive.

Monilethrix is characterized clinically by fragile scalp hair shafts and diffuse perifollicular papules with erythema. As the hair of affected individuals with monilethrix is easily broken, they frequently show sparse hair (hypotrichosis). In most cases, monilethrix shows an autosomal dominant inheritance pattern (MIM 158000), while autosomal recessive forms (MIM 252200) also exist. Under microscopy, the hair shaft of affected individuals with monilethrix dysplays a characteristic anomaly, known as beaded or moniliform hair, which shows periodic changes in hair diameter. As a result, the hair leads to the formation of nodes and internodes (Figure 5) [12]. Autosomal dominant form of the disease is caused by heterozygous mutations in *KRT81*, *KRT83*, and *KRT86* genes, which encode type II hair keratins K81, K83, and K86, respectively [13, 14]. All the mutations identified to date result in a deleterious amino acid substitution within either the HIM or the HTM of the rod domain. These hair keratins are predominantly expressed in the keratinizing zone of the hair shaft cortex (Figure 6) [15]. Although precise mechanisms to cause moniliform hair remain elusive, mutations in these hair keratin genes are predicted to result in disruption of the KIF formation, leading to an abnormal hair shaft keratinization.

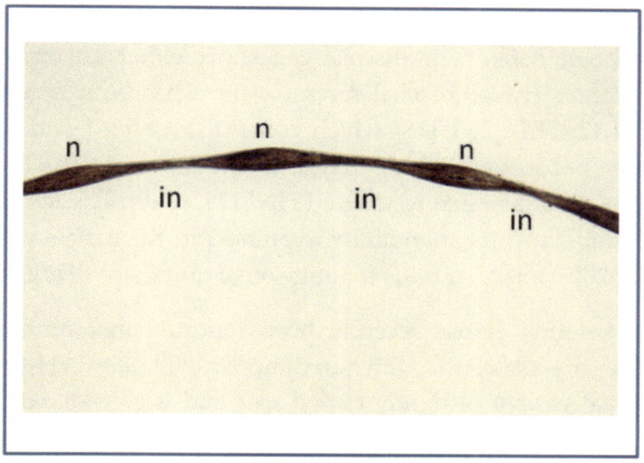

Figure 5. Moniliform hair. N, node; in, internode.

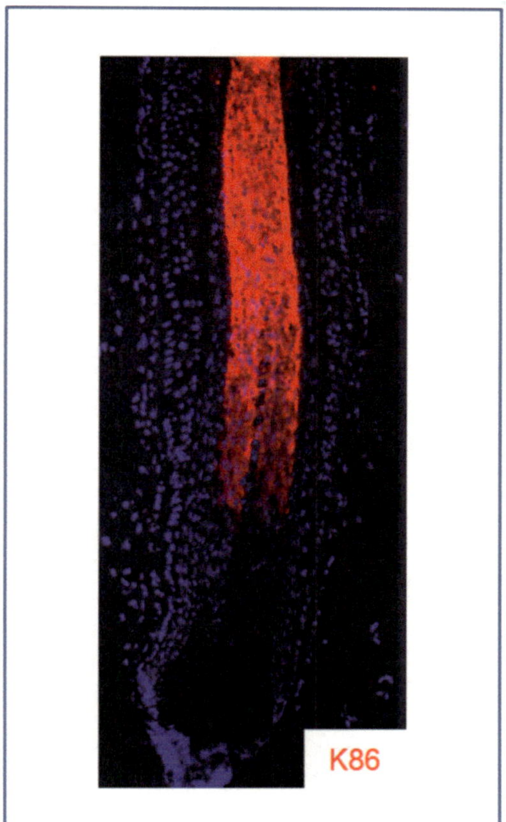

Figure 6. Expression of hair keratin K86 in the human hair shaft cortex.

Pure hair and nail ectodermal dysplasia (PHNED; MIM 602032) is characterized by absent or sparse hair, as well as nail dystrophy [16]. Hairs of affected individuals with PHNED are short and thin, and perifollicular papules can also be observed. In addition, their nails typically show koilonychia (spoon nails). The disease can show either an autosomal dominant or recessive inheritance trait. The autosomal recessive form has been mapped to chromosome 17p12-q21.2 [17] and 12p11.1-q21.1 [18] which contain the type I and type II keratin gene clusters, respectively. Subsequently, homozygous mutations in *KRT85* gene have been identified in families with autosomal recessive PHNED [18, 19]. The *KRT85* gene encodes the type II hair keratin K85, which is abundantly expressed in the matrix region of both the HF and the nail units [15, 20]. Molecular basis for autosomal dominant PHNED is yet unknown.

In addition to hair keratins, it has recently been reported that mutations in HF-specific epithelial keratin genes are associated with hereditary woolly hair (WH)/hypotrichosis. WH is defined as an abnormal variant of tightly curled hair and is considered to be a kind of hair growth deficiency [21]. There are both syndromic and non-syndromic forms of WH. The non-syndromic forms of WH can show either an autosomal-dominant (ADWH; MIM 194300) or -recessive (ARWH; MIM 278150) inheritance pattern. It is well-known that WH is frequently associated with hypotrichosis. Recently, heterozygous mutations in *KRT74* and *KRT71* genes have been identified in families with ADWH/hypotrichosis (Figure 7) [22-24]. Importantly, the *KRT74* and the *KRT71* genes encode the IRS-specific type II epithelial keratins K74 and K71, respectively (Figure 8) [25]. It can be postulated that disruption of the KIF formation in the IRS results in a failure to guide the hair growth, and leads to WH phenotype. Interestingly, *KRT71* mutations have also been identified in mice, rats, cats, and dogs, all of which show wavy coat phenotypes [26-30]. These data strongly suggest crucial roles of the IRS-specific epithelial keratins in the HF development and hair growth across mammalian species.

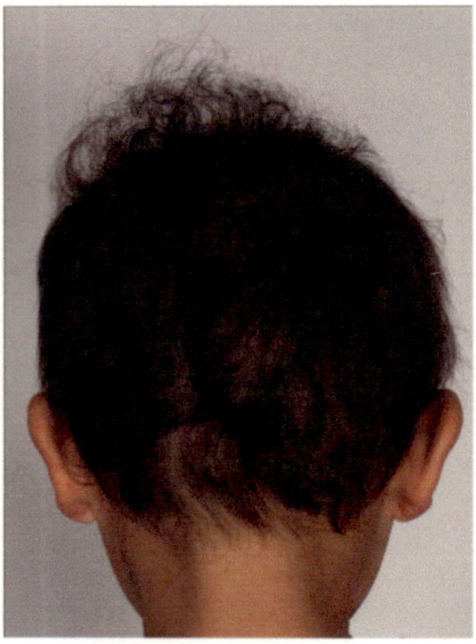

Figure 7. Clinical features of autosomal dominant woolly hair/hypotrichosis caused by a mutation in the *KRT71* gene.

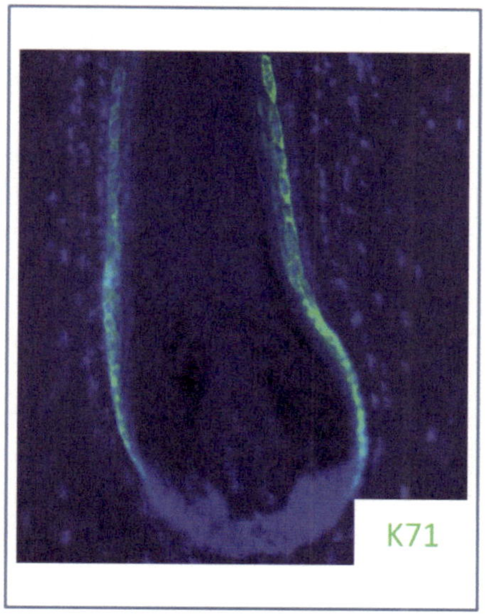

Figure 8. Expression of the IRS-specific karatin K71 in the human hair follicle.

4. Hereditary hair disorders resulting from disruption of cell-cell adhesion molecules

Similar to epidermis, the HF epithelium possess a number of cell-cell adhesion structures, such as desmosomes, corneodesmosomes, adherens junctions, gap junctions, and tight junctions, which play important roles in maintaining the structure and the function of the HF. It has been shown that disruption of any of these structures can result in hereditary hair disorders in humans (Table 2).

Desmosome is a critical structure for cell-cell adhesion in most epithelial tissues, including the HF. The major structural component of the desmosome is the desmosomal cadherin family, which is comprised of the desmogleins (DSGs) and desmocollins (DSCs). In humans, 4 *DSG* genes (*DSG1-DSG4*) and 3 *DSC* genes (*DSC1-DSC3*) are located on chromosome 18q12. These desmosomal cadherin family members are glycoproteins with single-pass transmembrane domain, and are involved in Ca^{2+}-dependent cell-cell adhesion, connecting with each other using their extracellular domains [31]. Within the cytoplasm, they interact with several other proteins, known as desmosomal plaque proteins, which include plakoglobin, plakophilin, and desmoplakin. The desmosomal plaque proteins contribute to anchor the KIF near the cell membrane. As such, the cell integrity and the cell-cell adhesion are maintained [31]. Recessively-inherited mutations in the *DSG4* gene have been shown to cause a non-syndromic form of hereditary hair disorder known as localized autosomal recessive hypotrichosis 1 (LAH1; MIM 607903) [32]. Affected individuals with LAH1 show sparse hairs on the scalp, chest, arms, and legs. The eyebrows and beard are less dense than normal, and the axillary hair, pubic hair, and eyelashes look normal in most cases. It is noteworthy that hair shafts of affected individuals with *DSG4* mutations are fragile and often show moniliform hair [33-35]. Therefore, the *DSG4* can also be regarded as a causative

disease	inheritance pattern	OMIM#	main symptoms	gene	protein, function
Localized autosomal recessive hypotrichosis 1 (LAH1)/monilethrix	AR	607903/ 252200	hypotrichosis, moniliform hair, perifollicular papules	*DSG4*	desmoglein 4
Hypotrichosis and recurrent skin vesicles	AR	613102	Hypotrichosis, skin vesicles or keratosis pilaris	*DSC3*	desmocollin 3
Naxos disease	AR	601214	WH, PPK, right ventricular cardiomyopathy	*JUP*	junctional plakoglobin
Carvajal syndrome	AR	605676	WH, PPK, left ventricular cardiomyopathy	*DSP*	desmoplakin
Ectodermal dysplasia/skin fragility syndrome	AR	604536	Hypotrichosis, fragile skin, nail dystrophy	*PKP1*	plakophilin 1
Hypotrichosis simplex of the scalp	AD	146520	Scalp-limited hypotrichosis	*CDSN*	corneodesmosin
Netherton syndrome	AR	256500	ichthyosiform erythroderma, atopic manifestation, bamboo hair	*SPINK5*	LEKTI (serine protease inhibitor)
Ichthyosis with hypotrichosis	AR	610765	ichthyosis, hypotrichosis	*ST14*	matriptase (serine protease)
Hypotrichosis with juvenile macular dystrophy	AR	601553	Hypotrichosis, weak eyesight	*CDH3*	P-cadherin
Ectodermal dysplasia, ectrodactyly, macular dystrophy (EEM) syndrome	AR	225280	Hypotrichosis, weak eyesight, ectrodactyly	*CDH3*	P-cadherin
Hidrotic ectodermal dysplasia (Clouston syndrome)	AD	129500	hypotrichosis, PPK, nail dystrophy	*GJB6*	connexin 30
Keratitis ichthyosis deafness (KID) syndrome	AD	148210	vascularizing keratitis, sensorial deafness, erythrokeratoderma, hypotrichosis	*GJB2* *GJB6*	connexin 26 connexin 30
Ichthyosis, leukocyte vacuoles, alopecia, and sclerosing cholangitis	AR	607626	Hypotrichosis, ichthyosis, jaundice, hapatomegaly,	*CLDN1*	claudin 1

AD, autosomal dominant; AR, autosomal recessive; WH, woolly hair; PPK, palmoplantar keratoderma.

Table 2. Hereditary hair disorders caused by disruption of cell-cell adhesion structures and the related molecules.

gene for autosomal recessive monilethrix. DSG4 is the only desmoglein member that is expressed in the hair shaft (Figure 9) [36], and its expression in the hair shaft cortex finely overlaps with K81, K83, and K86, of which mutations cause autosomal dominant monilethrix. More recently, a homozygous nonsense mutation in the *DSC3* gene has been identified in a family with an autosomal recessive form of hypotrichosis [37]. The disease is characterized by sparse scalp hairs and small vesicle formation on the scalp and extremities (hypotrichosis and recurrent skin vesicles; MIM 613102) [37], while there is an argument that the vesicles may be keratosis pilaris [38]. In addition, mutations in genes encoding desmosomal plaque proteins can also show hair phenotypes (Table 2). For example, mutations in junctional plakoglobin (*JUP*) and desmoplakin (*DSP*) genes are known to underlie Naxos disease (MIM 601214) and Carvajal syndrome (MIM 605676), respectively [39, 40]. Both diseases show an autosomal recessive inheritance pattern and are characterized by woolly hair, palmoplantar keratoderma, and severe cardiomyopathy. Furthermore, loss of function mutations in plakophilin 1 (*PKP1*) gene cause a rare autosomal recessive disease named ectodermal dysplasia/skin fragility syndrome (MIM 604536) [41].

Corneodesmosome is a modified desmosome in the stratum corneum (SC) of the epidermis, and plays a crucial in the desquamation process. One of the major components of the corneodesmosome is corneodesmosin (CDSN). CDSN is secreted by cytoplasmic vesicles into the extracellular core of desmosomes, and is progressively proteolysed by several serine

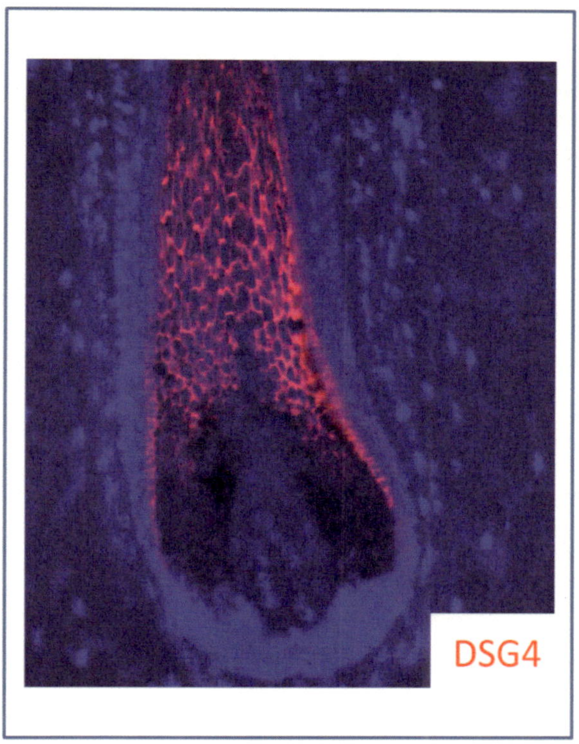

Figure 9. Expression of desmoglein 4 (DSG4) in the human hair shaft.

proteases, such as kallikrein-related peptidases, which leads to the loss of cell-cell adhesivity in the SC and causes desquamation [42]. CDSN is also expressed predominantly in the IRS of the HF, and thus is considered to be important for terminal differentiation, as well as subsequent degradation of the IRS [43]. In 2003, heterozygous nonsense mutations in the *CDSN* gene have been identified in patients with hereditary hypotrichosis simplex of the scalp (HHSS; MIM 146520), which is an autosomal dominant disorder characterized by sparse hairs limited to the scalp region without any obvious hair shaft anomalies (Figure 10) [44]. Histologically, the IRS of the patients' HF was disturbed, which was consistent with the expression of CDSN in the IRS. Furthermore, aggregates of abnormal CDSN were detected around the HF, as well as in the papillary dermis in patients' skin [44]. These aggregates have recently been shown to be an amyloid protein derived from the mutant CDSN, which is likely to be toxic to the HF cells [45]. Therefore, the mutant CDSN protein appears to function in a dominant negative manner, affect growth of the HF, and lead to HHSS. In addition to HHSS, it has been reported that mutations in other genes functionally related with CDSN can show some hair phenotypes associated with congenital ichthyosis. Of these, Netherton syndrome (NS; MIM 256500) is a rare autosomal recessive condition characterized by ichthyosiform erythroderma, atopic manifestation, and the hair shaft anomaly, known as bamboo hair (trichorrhexis invaginata) (Figure 11). The NS is caused by loss of function mutations in *SPINK5* gene which encodes a serine protease inhibitor named LEKTI (lymphoepithelial Kazal-type-related inhibitor) [46]. Disruption of LEKTI has been shown to result in upregulation of serine proteases and excess desquamation due to premature proteolysis of CDSN [47, 48]. Furthermore, it has been reported that recessively-inherited mutations in *ST14* gene, which encodes a member of serine proteases (matriptase), underlie ichthyosis with hypotrichosis syndrome (MIM 610765) [49]. Sum of these genetic data suggest that balanced expression of CDSN, serine proteases, and their inhibitors is critical for the HF differentiation.

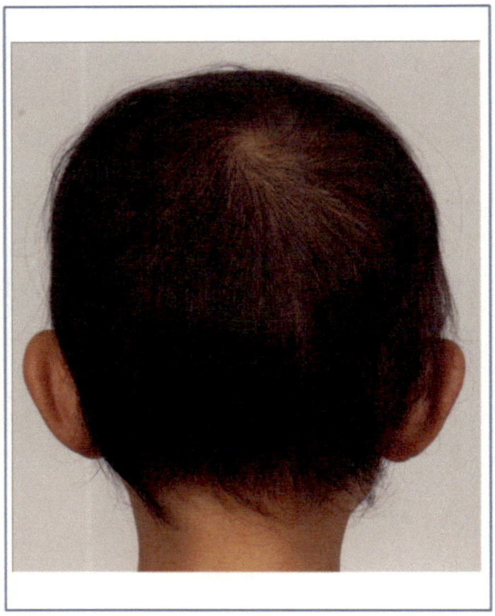

Figure 10. Clinical features of hypotrichosis simplex of the scalp.

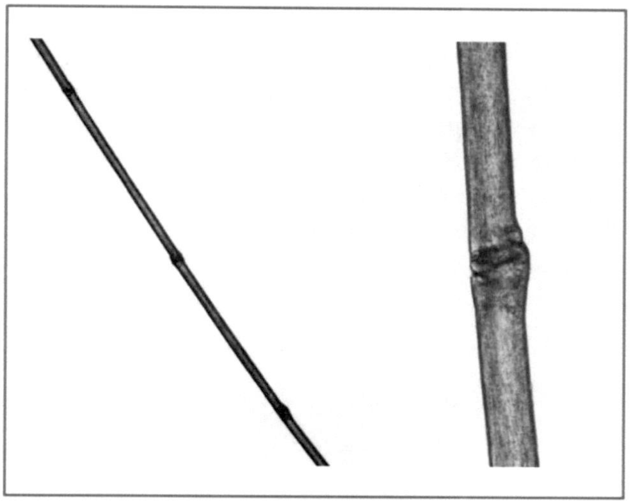

Figure 11. Bamboo hair (trichorrhexis invaginata).

E- and P-cadherins are classical cadherins which are a major component of adherens junctions in the HF. When the HF placode is formed during embryogenesis, the expression of E-cadherin is markedly downregulated, while P-cadherin is simultaneously upregulated, and prominant expression of P-cadherin persists in the proximal portion of the HF. This phenomenon, known as cadherin switching, is believed to be essential for the HF morphogenesis [50]. In addition, P-cadherin has recently been shown to be important for postnatal hair growth and cycling as well [51]. The critical role of these classical cadherins in the HF has been further supported by two hereditary diseases resulting from mutations in the P-cadherin gene (*CDH3*). First, mutations in the *CDH3* gene are known to underlie hypotrichosis with juvenile macular dystrophy (HJMD; MIM 601553), which is an autosomal recessive disease characterized by sparse hair and weak eyesight due to macular dystrophy of the retina [52]. In addition, it has been reported that another disease, ectodermal dysplasia, ectrodactyly and macular dystrophy (EEM syndrome; MIM 225280), is also caused by recessively-inherited mutations in the *CDH3* gene [53]. Affected individuals with EEM syndrome show common hair and eye phenotype with HJMD. However, EEM patients also shows split hand/foot malformation (ectrodactyly), suggesting crucial roles of P-cadherin in the development of not only hair and retina, but also the limbs in humans. There are no clear genotype-phenotype correlations in *CDH3* mutations, as it has been reported that a same mutation in the *CDH3* gene caused HJMD in one family [54], while EEM syndrome in another family [53]. Identification of modifier gene(s) may reveal this paradox in the future.

Gap junction (GJ) is a specialized intercellular structure that provides a pathway for both metabolic and ionic coupling between adjacent cells and maintains tissue homeostasis [55]. Connexins (Cxs) are 4-pass transmembrane proteins and the major component of the GJs. Clouston syndrome (MIM 129500), also known as hidrotic ectodermal dysplasia, is an autosomal dominant condition characterized by hypotrichosis, nail dystrophy, and palmoplantar keratoderma. The disease is caused by mutations in *GJB6* gene which encodes Cx30 [56]. In addition, mutations in *GJB2* gene encoding Cx26 are known to underlie keratitis-ichthyosis-deafness syndrome (KID; MIM 148210) [57]. The triad of KID is vascularizing keratitis, profound sensorial hearing loss, and erythrokeratoderma. Additionally, patients with KID show severe hypotrichosis in high frequency. Interestingly, it has been reported that a mutation in the *GJB6* gene (V37E) can show phenotypes resembling KID [58]. These Cx proteins are mainly expressed in the ORS of the HF (Figure 12) [59, 60], and thus they may play some roles in maintaining the function of the HF stem cells.

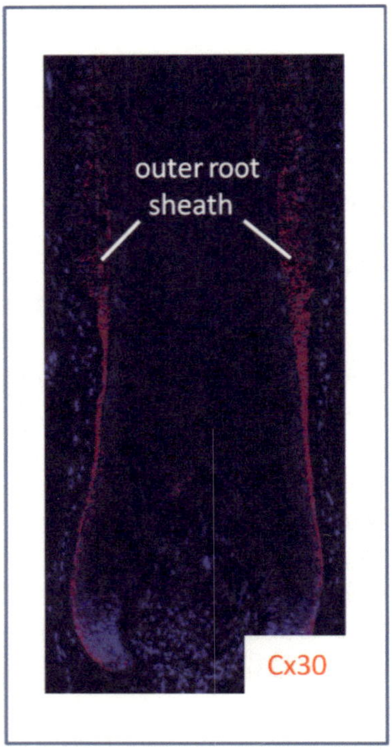

Figure 12. Cx30 expression in the human hair follicle.

In addition to the cell-cell adhesion structures described above, tight junction (TJ) also exists in the HF epithelium and expression patterns of TJ-associated proteins in the HF have previously been characterized [61]. Disruption of *CLDN1* gene encoding claudin 1, a major structural component of TJ, has recently been shown to cause a severe autosomal recessive syndrome, known as ichthyosis, leukocyte vacuoles, alopecia, and sclerosing cholangitis (MIM 607626) [62].

5. Hereditary hair disorders associated with transcription factors

During the past 20 years, numerous genes that are expressed in the HF have been identified, and various transcription factors have been shown to be involved in transcriptional regulation of these genes. Of these, p63 is one of the main transcription factors expressed in the HF. During the HF morphogenesis, p63 is abundantly expressed in the HF placode (Figure 13). In the postnatal stage, it is strongly expressed in the ORS and the matrix region of the HF (Figure 14). It has previously been reported that mutations in *TP63* gene encoding p63 cause several autosomal dominant diseases including ectodermal dysplasia, ectrodactyly, cleft lip/palate (EEC) syndrome (MIM 604292), ankyloblepharon, ectodermal defects, and cleft lip/palate (AEC) syndrome (MIM 106260) and Rapp-Hodgkin syndrome (MIM 129400) (Table 3) [63-65]. In most cases, patients with these syndromes result in scarring alopecia, and their hair shafts are coarse and twisted (Figure 15). It is noteworthy that affected individuals with *TP63* mutations show large phenotypic overlaps in hair and limbs with P-cadherin (*CDH3*) mutations. p63 colocalizes with P-cadherin in developing HF placode and limb buds during mouse embryogenesis. Importantly, it has been demonstrated that the *CDH3* is a direct target gene of p63 [66].

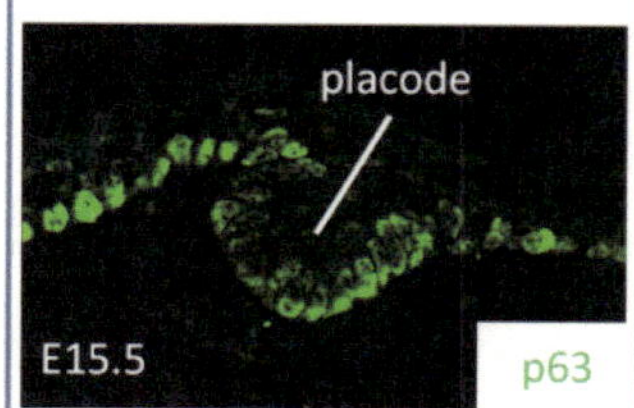

Figure 13. P63 expression in the developing mouse hair follicle placode.

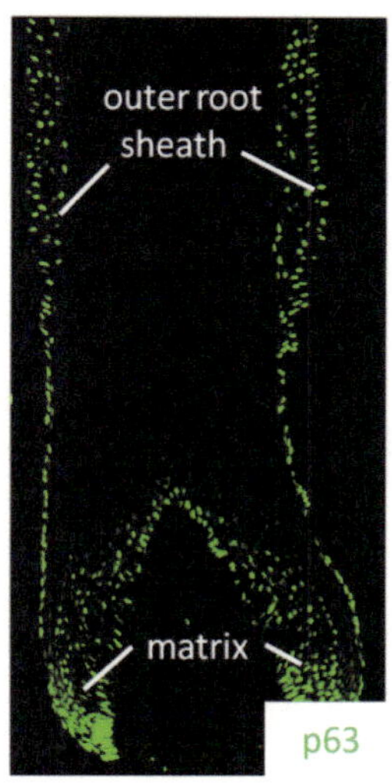

Figure 14. p63 expression in the human hair follicle.

disease	inheritance pattern	OMIM#	main symptoms	gene	Protein, function
Ectrodactyly, ectodermal dysplasia, and cleft lip/palate (EEC) syndrome	AD	604292	hypotrichosis, ectrodactyly, cleft lip/palate, hypodontia	*TP63*	tumor protein p63
Ankyloblepharon, ectodermal defects, and cleft lip/palate (AEC) syndrome	AD	106260	hypotrichosis, ankyloblepharon, skin erosion, cleft lip/palate, hypodontia	*TP63*	tumor protein p63
Rapp-Hodgkin syndrome	AD	129400	hypotrichosis, cleft lip/palate, hypodontia	*TP63*	tumor protein p63
T cell immunodeficiency, congenital alopecia, and nail dystrophy (human nude phenotype)	AR	601705	atrichia, nail dystrophy, T-cell immuodeficiency	*FOXN1*	Forkhead box N1
Atrichia with papular lesions	AR	209500	atrichia, papules	*HR*	Hair less (transcriptional corepressor)
Marie-Unna hereditary hypotrichosis	AD	146550	Hypotrichosis, wiry hair	*U2HR*	Small peptide that regulates translation of the HR protein
Trichorhinophalangeal syndrome type I/type III	AD	190350/190351	Hypotrichosis, peer-shaped nose, brachydactyly, clinodactyly	*TRPS1*	Zing finger transcription factor
Hypotrichosis-lymphedema-telangiectasia syndrome	AD/AR	607823	Hypotrichosis, lymphedema, telangiectasia (easily visible blood vessels)	*SOX18*	SRY-BOX 18
Trichodontoosseous syndrome	AD	190320	WH, hypodontia, bone anomalies	*DLX3*	Distal-less homeobox 3

AD, autosomal dominant; AR, autosomal recessive; WH, woolly hair.

Table 3. Hereditary hair disorders resulting from mutations in transcription factors.

FOXN1, also known as WHN, is a transcription factor expressed in the matrix and the hair shaft of the HF, and has been shown to regulate the expression of several hair keratin genes [67]. FOXN1 is expressed in not only the HF, but also in the nail units and thymus. Mutations in the *FOXN1* gene have been reported to underlie T-cell immunodeficiency, congenital alopecia, and nail dystrophy (MIM 601705), which is an autosomal recessive disease and represents the human counterpart of the nude mouse phenotype, suggesting the crucial roles of FOXN1 in development of skin appendages, as well as thymus in both humans and mice [68].

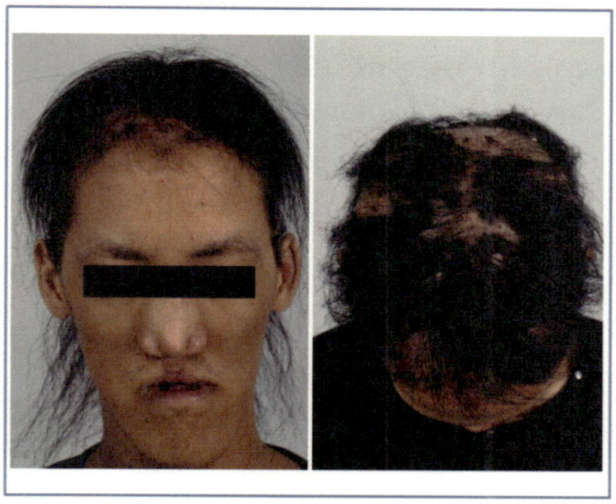

Figure 15. Clinical features of Rapp-Hodgkin syndrome.

Hairless (*HR*) is a putative single zinc-finger transcription factor which is known to regulate the catagen phase of the hair cycle [69]. Recessively-inherited mutations in the *HR* gene have been shown to underlie atrichia with popular lesions (APL; MIM 209500) [70]. APL is characterized by early onset of generalized complete hair loss (atrichia), which is followed by papular eruptions due to formation of dermal cyst after an abnormal first catagen phase [71]. Mutations responsible for APL have been found in coding exons or exon-intron boundary sequences of the *HR* gene, all of which were predicted to result in loss of expression and/or function of the HR protein. Recently, another disease, known as Marie-Unna hypotrichosis (MUH; MIM 146550), has been shown to be associated with the *HR* gene. MUH is a non-syndromic hereditary hair disorder showing an autosomal dominant inheritance pattern. Affected individuals with MUH typically exhibit sparse scalp and facial hair at birth. Subsequently, coarse, wiry, and twisted hairs develop in early childhood. Hair loss progresses with aging, which leads to a complete alopecia or a phenotype just like androgenetic alopecia. MUH was previously mapped to the *HR* locus on chromosome 8p21.3 [72]. However, direct sequencing analysis of coding sequences of the *HR* gene failed to detect mutations. Later on, Wen et al. found that the promoter region of the *HR* gene has four potential upstream open reading frames (uORFs), which were designated *U1HR-U4HR*. Strikingly, direct sequencing analysis of the *U1HR-U4HR* in patients with MUH has led to the identification of mutations within the *U2HR* sequences, which encode a small peptide of 34 amino acid residues [73]. *In vitro* studies have suggested that this small peptide encoded by the *U2HR* downregulates the *HR* expression at the translational level, and loss-of-function mutations in the *U2HR* results in overexpression of the HR protein [73]. Besides these findings, actual consequences resulting from *U2HR* mutations *in vivo* remain elusive.

TRPS1 is a transcription factor with GATA-type and Ikaros-type zinc finger domains, which has been shown to be abundantly expressed in both epithelial and mesenchymal components in the developing mouse HFs [74]. Furthermore, it has recently been reported that Trps1 plays crucial roles in regulating the expression of several Wnt inhibitors and various transcription factors during vibrissa follicle morphogenesis in mice [75]. In humans, mutations in the *TRPS1* gene are known to cause trichorhinophalangeal syndrome type I (TRPS I; MIM 190350) or type III (TRPS III; MIM 190351), both of which show an autosomal dominant inheritance trait, and are characterized by sparse hair and a number of craniofacial and skeletal abnormalities, such as peer-shaped nose and brachydactyly. Hypotrichosis is the most prominent in the temporal region of the scalp (Figure 16) [76, 77].

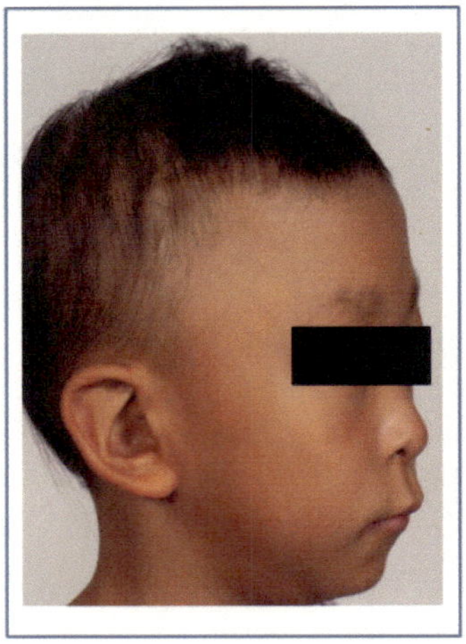

Figure 16. Clinical features of TRPS I.

In addition to the transcription factors described above, several other members are also associated with hereditary hair diseases. For instance, both dominantly- and recessively-inherited mutations in *SOX18* gene underlie hypotrichosis-lymphedema-telangiectasia syndrome (MIM 607823) [78] and dominantly-inherited mutations in *DLX3* gene cause trichodontoosseous syndrome (MIM 190320), respectively (Table 3) [79].

6. Hereditary hair disorders caused by disruption in signaling pathways

It has been shown via analyses using mice models that several signaling pathways play crucial roles in the HF morphogenesis and development. In humans, disruption of these signaling pathways has been demonstrated to underlie various hereditary hair disorders (Table 4). In addition, information obtained from the analysis of hereditary hair diseases has highlighted a novel signaling pathway that had not previously been known to play a role in the HF development.

Hypohidrotic ectodermal dysplasia (HED), also known as Christ-Siemens-Touraine syndrome, is a rare genetic disease characterized by abnormal development of hair, teeth, and sweat glands. Most cases of HED show an X-linked recessive inheritance pattern (MIM 305100), while a minority of HED is inherited as either an autosomal dominant (MIM 129490) or an autosomal recessive trait (MIM 224900). During the last 15 years, the molecular basis for HED has gradually been disclosed. X-linked HED is caused by mutations in ectodysplasin (*EDA*) gene [80], and autosomal forms of HED are resulting from mutations in either EDA-receptor (*EDAR*) [81] or EDAR-associated death domain

disease	inheritance pattern	OMIM#	main symptoms	gene	protein, function
Hypohidrotic ectodermal dysplasia	XR	305100	Hypotrichosis, hypohidrosis, hypodontia	EDA	ectodysplasin A1 (EDA-A1)
	AD	129490		EDAR EDARADD TRAF6	EDA-A1 receptor EDAR-associated death domain TNF receptor-associated factor 6
	AR	224900		EDAR EDARADD	EDA-A1 receptor EDAR-associated death domain
Odontoonychodermal dysplasia	AR	257980	Hypotrichosis, hypodontia, nail dystrophy, PPK	WNT10A	Wnt ligand
Generalized hereditary hypotrichosis simplex	AD	605389	hypotrichosis	APCDD1	Wnt inhibitor
Localized autosomal recessive hypotrichosis 2 (LAH2)/autosomal recessive woolly hair 2 (ARWH2)	AR	604379	WH, hypotrichosis	LIPH	phosphatidic acid-selective phospholipase A1α (PA-PLA1α)
LAH3/ARWH1	AR	611452/278150	WH, hypotrichosis	LPAR6	LPA6 (LPA receptor)
Inflammatory skin and bowel disease	AR	614328	erythema, diarrhea, WH	ADAM17	Tumor necrosis factor converting enzyme (TACE)

XR, X-linked recessive; AD, autosomal dominant; AR, autosomal recessive; PPK, palmoplantar keratoderma; LPA, lysophosphatidic acid.

Table 4. Hereditary hair disorders associated with disruption of signaling pathways.

(*EDARADD*) [82] genes. The *EDA* gene encodes several isoforms of a type II transmembrane protein via alternative splicing [83]. Of these, ectodysplasin-A1 (EDA-A1) is the longest isoform which belongs to the tumor necrosis factor (TNF) ligand superfamily. EDAR, the receptor of EDA-A1 [84], is a type I transmembrane protein and a member of the TNF receptor superfamily with a potential death domain in its intracellular region. During the development of ectoderm-derived organs, EDA-A1 binds to its receptor EDAR, which subsequently associates with its adaptor EDARADD. Additionally, EDARADD protein interacts with TNF receptor-associated factor 6 (TRAF6), which further forms a complex with TGFβ-activated kinase 1 (TAK1) and TAK1-binding protein 2 (TAB2) within the cytoplasm, leading to activate the downstream NF-κB [85]. Most recently, a heterozygous mutation in the *TRAF6* gene has been identified in a patient showing typical clinical features of HED [86]. Since EDA-A1, EDAR, EDARADD, and TRAF6 are closely related to each other in a signaling pathway, mutations in any of these four pathway components result in identical phenotypic characteristics among patients.

Odontoonychodermal dysplasia (OODD; MIM 257980) is an autosomal recessive disease which is characterized by various ectodermal abnormalities including hypotrichosis, hypodontia, nail dystrophy, and palmoplantar keratoderma. It has recently been shown that OODD is caused by loss of function mutations in the *WNT10A* gene, which encodes a WNT ligand [87]. It is noted that some affected individuals with *WNT10A* mutations can show phenotypes resembling HED [88], indicating the close relationship between EDA-A1/EDAR signaling and Wnt signaling, which has also been suggested by experiments in mice models [89].

In addition to Wnt ligands, abnormal function of Wnt inhibitors has recently been shown to cause a hereditary hair disorder in humans. Generalized hypotrichosis simplex (GHS; MIM 605389) is an autosomal dominant non-syndromic hair disorder which is characterized by progressive loss of scalp and body hairs starting in the middle of the first decade of life and almost complete baldness by the third decade [90]. In several families with GHS, an identical heterozygous missense mutation (L9R) has been identified in *APCDD1* gene on chromosome 18p11.22 [91, 92]. The *APCDD1* gene encodes a single-pass transmembrane protein which is abundantly expressed in the dermal papilla, the matrix and the hair shaft of human HF. Functional studies in cultured cells, chick embryos, and xenopus have revealed that APCDD1 inhibits Wnt signaling potentially via interacting Wnt ligands and their co-receptors LRPs [91]. In addition, it has been demonstrated that the L9R-mutant APCDD1 protein functions in a dominant negative manner against wild-type APCDD1 protein [91]. Therefore, Wnt activity is predicted to be upregulated in patients' HFs. It is postulated that chronic stimulation by Wnt signaling may result in depletion of stem cell pool in the HF bulge, leading to GHS.

Recently, a signaling of lipid mediators has been shown to play essential roles in hair growth. About a decade ago, phosphatidic acid, has been demonstrated to promote hair growth in organ culture system, suggesting a potential role of lipids in hair growth [93]. Later on, it has been reported that mutations in lipase H (*LIPH*) gene underlies an autosomal recessively-inherited hypotrichosis (Localized autosomal recessive hypotrichosis 2 (LAH2); MIM 604379) [94]. Affected individuals with LAH2 show sparse hair on their scalp and extremities, whereas facial and sexual hairs look normal. In addition, it is noteworthy that patients with *LIPH* mutations show woolly hair (WH) in high frequency (Figure 17) [95], thus the *LIPH* can be regarded as a causative gene responsible for autosomal recessive WH (ARWH). Most affected individuals with *LIPH* mutations showed mainly WH during early childhood, and then exhibited wide variability in the hypotrichosis phenotype with aging [96].

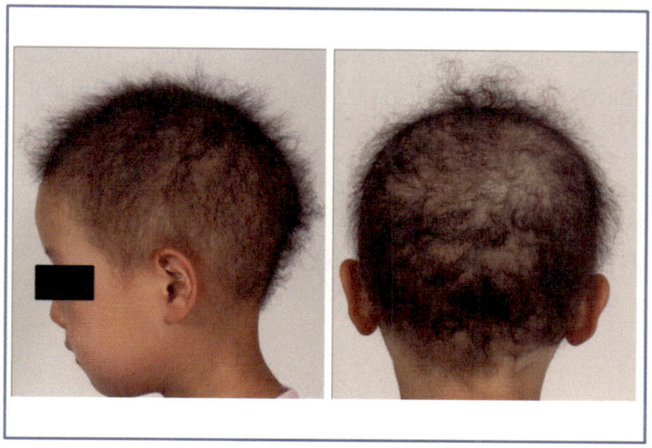

Figure 17. Clinical features of LAH2/woolly hair caused by mutations in the *LIPH* gene.

The *LIPH* gene encodes cell membrane-associated phosphatidic acid-selective phospholipase $A_1\alpha$ (PA-$PLA_1\alpha$) which produces 2-acyl lysophosphatidic acid (LPA) from phosphatidic acid [97]. As LPA activates cells through binding with its receptor, the existence of LPA receptor(s) in the HF had been expected, which has been idenitified by the analyses of additional families with ARWH/hypotrichosis without carrying mutations in the *LIPH* gene. Affected individuals in these families showed WH and associated hypotrichosis (Localized autosomal recessive hypotrichosis 3 (LAH3); MIM611452), which were almost identical phenotypes to those with *LIPH* mutations. Linkage studies and positional cloning have led to the identification of mutations in *LPAR6* gene, also known as *P2RY5*, in these families [98, 99]. The *LPAR6* gene encodes a G protein-coupled receptor LPA_6 (P2Y5), which has clearly been proved to be a receptor of LPA [100]. Both PA-$PLA_1\alpha$ and LPA_6 are mainly expressed in the IRS of human HF [24, 99]. Importantly, their expression overlaps with K71 and K74, of which mutations underlie autosomal dominant WH/hypotrichosis. Sum of these data strongly suggest the crucial roles of PA-$PLA_1\alpha$/LPA/LPA_6 pathway in the HF differentiation and hair growth, and its downstream signaling may be involved in regulating expression of the IRS-specific keratins. More recently, significant findings have been reported, which have revealed the downstream signaling of the PA-$PLA_1\alpha$/LPA/LPA_6 pathway. Inoue et al. have produced *Liph*-knockout (KO) mice which exhibited a wavy coat phenotype resembling WH in humans [101]. In addition, a series of expression studies in the mutant mice, as well as detailed *in vitro* analyses, have demonstrated that the PA-$PLA_1\alpha$/LPA/LPA_6 axis regulates differentiation and maturation of mouse HF via a signaling pathway composed of tumor necrosis factor converting enzyme (TACE), transforming growth facor (TGF)-α, and epidermal growth factor receptor (EGFR) [101]. It has been shown that LPA produced by PA-$PLA_1\alpha$ stimulated its receptor LPA_6, which subsequently activated TACE. Then, TACE induced ectodomain shedding of TGF-α, which resulted in transactivation of EGFR (Figure 18) [101]. Notably, in the HF of the *Liph*-KO mice, the expression of cleaved TGF-α, tyrosine-phosphorylated EGFR, LPA, and the IRS-specific K71, were significantly reduced [101]. Most recently, a recessively-inherited mutation in *ADAM17* gene encoding TACE have been shown to cause inflammatory skin and bowel disease (MIM 614328) in humans, and affected individuals with the *ADAM17* mutation appear to show WH phenotypes, similar to patients with *LIPH* or *LPAR6* mutations [102]. These findings strongly suggest that the PA-PLA$_1\alpha$/LPA/LPA$_6$ signaling can be involved in activating TACE in humans as well.

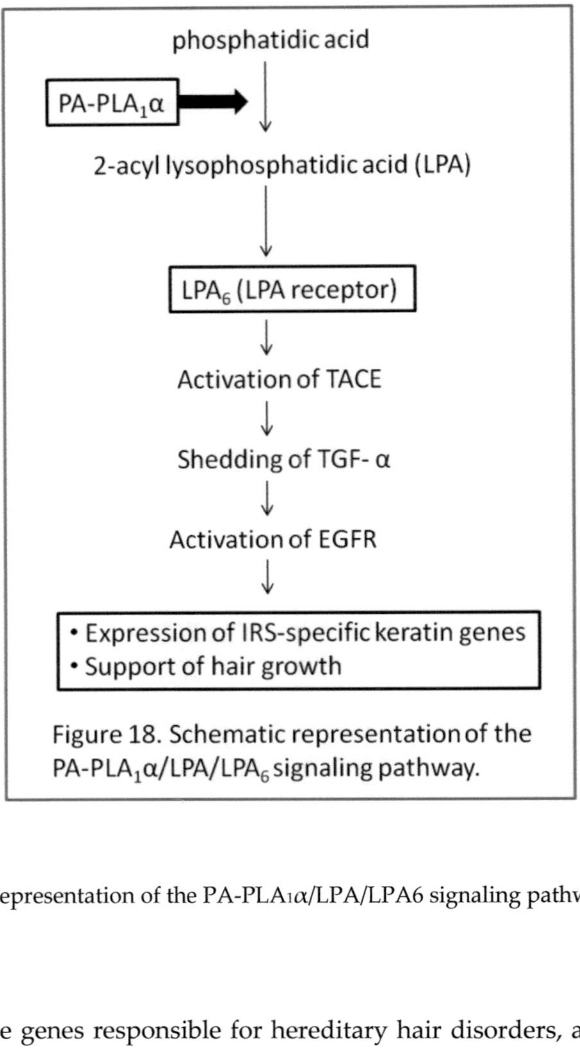

Figure 18. Schematic representation of the PA-PLA$_1\alpha$/LPA/LPA6 signaling pathway.

7. Conclusions

To identify causative genes responsible for hereditary hair disorders, as well as to disclose the functional relationship between these genes, has provided precious information to better understand the complex mechanisms for the HF development and cycling in humans. It is highly expected that recently-established methods in molecular genetics, especially whole genome sequencing [103], will enable us to find additional causative genes for the diseases. These genes may be associated with not only rare hair disorders, but also determining the hair texture in healthy individuals and/or more common hair diseases, such as alopecia areata and androgenetic alopecia.

Author details

Yutaka Shimomura

Laboratory of Genetic Skin Diseases, Niigata University Graduate School of Medical and Dental Sciences, Niigata, Japan

Acknowledgement

I appreciate Drs. Atsushi Fujimoto and Hiroki Fujikawa (Niigata University, Japan) for their assistance to make figures. This work was supported in part by the Special Coordination Funds for Promoting Science and Technology from the Ministry of Education, Culture, Sports, Science and Technology of Japan (MEXT) to Y.S.

8. References

[1] Millar SE. Molecular mechanisms regulating hair follicle development. J Invest Dermatol. 2002;118(2): 216-25.

[2] Shimomura Y, Christiano AM. Biology and genetics of hair. Annu Rev Genomics Hum Genet. 2010;11: 109-32.

[3] Cotsarelis G, Sun TT, Lavker RM. Label-retaining cells reside in the bulge area of pilosebaceous unit: implications for follicular stem cells, hair cycle, and skin carcinogenesis. Cell. 1990;61(7): 1329-37.

[4] Oshima H, Rochat A, Kedzia C, Kobayashi K, Barrandon Y. Morphogenesis and renewal of hair follicles from adult multipotent stem cells. Cell. 2001;104(2): 233-45.

[5] Coulombe PA, Omary MB. 'Hard' and 'soft' principles defining the structure, function and regulation of keratin intermediate filaments. Curr Opin Cell Biol. 2002;14(1): 110-22.

[6] Shimomura Y, Ito M. Human hair keratin-associated proteins. J Investig Dermatol Symp Proc. 2005;10(3):230-3.

[7] Rogers MA, Langbein L, Praetzel-Wunder S, Winter H, Schweizer J. Human hair keratin-associated proteins (KAPs). Int Rev Cytol. 2006;251: 209-63.

[8] Rogers MA, Winter H, Wolf C, Heck M, Schweizer J. Characterization of a 190-kilobase pair domain of human type I hair keratin genes. J Biol Chem. 1998;273(41): 26683-91.

[9] Rogers MA, Winter H, Langbein L, Wolf C, Schweizer J. Characterization of a 300 kbp region of human DNA containing the type II hair keratin gene domain. J Invest Dermatol. 2000;114(3): 464-72.

[10] Moll R, Divo M, Langbein L. The human keratins: biology and pathology. Histochem Cell Biol. 2008;129(6): 705-33.

[11] Langbein L, Yoshida H, Praetzel-Wunder S, Parry DA, Schweizer J. The keratins of the human beard hair medulla: the riddle in the middle. J Invest Dermatol. 2010;130(1): 55-73.

[12] Ito M, Hashimoto K, Yorder FW. Monilethrix: an ultrastructural study. J Cutan Pathol. 1984;11(6): 513-21.

[13] Winter H, Rogers MA, Langbein L, Stevens HP, Leigh IM, Labrèze C, Roul S, Taieb A, Krieg T, Schweizer J. Mutations in the hair cortex keratin hHb6 cause the inherited hair disease monilethrix. Nat Genet. 1997;16(4): 372-4.

[14] van Steensel MA, Steijlen PM, Bladergroen RS, Vermeer M, van Geel M. A missense mutation in the type II hair keratin hHb3 is associated with monilethrix. J Med Genet. 2005;42(3): e19.

[15] Langbein L, Rogers MA, Winter H, Praetzel S, Schweizer J. The catalog of human hair keratins. II. Expression of the six type II members in the hair follicle and the combined catalog of human type I and II keratins. J Biol Chem. 2001;276(37): 35123-32.

[16] Barbareschi M, Cambiaghi S, Crupi AC, Tadini G. Family with "pure" hair-nail ectodermal dysplasia. Am J Med Genet. 1997;72(1): 91-3.

[17] Naeem M, Jelani M, Lee K, Ali G, Chishti MS, Wali A, Gul A, John P, Hassan MJ, Leal SM, Ahmad W. Ectodermal dysplasia of hair and nail type: mapping of a novel locus to chromosome 17p12-q21.2. Br J Dermatol. 2006;155(6): 1184-90.

[18] Naeem M, Wajid M, Lee K, Leal SM, Ahmad W. A mutation in the hair matrix and cuticle keratin KRTHB5 gene causes ectodermal dysplasia of hair and nail type. J Med Genet. 2006;43(3): 274-9.

[19] Shimomura Y, Wajid M, Kurban M, Sato N, Christiano AM. Mutations in the keratin 85 (KRT85/hHb5) gene underlie pure hair and nail ectodermal dysplasia. J Invest Dermatol. 2010;130(3): 892-5.

[20] Perrin C, Langbein L, Schweizer J. Expression of hair keratins in the adult nail unit: an immunohistochemical analysis of the onychogenesis in the proximal nail fold, matrix and nail bed. Br J Dermatol. 2004;151(2): 362-71.

[21] Chien AJ, Valentine MC, Sybert VP. Hereditary woolly hair and keratosis pilaris. J Am Acad Dermatol. 2006;54(2 Suppl): S35-9.

[22] Shimomura Y, Wajid M, Petukhova L, Kurban M, Christiano AM. Autosomal-dominant woolly hair resulting from disruption of keratin 74 (KRT74), a potential determinant of human hair texture. Am J Hum Genet. 2010;86(4): 632-8.

[23] Wasif N, Naqvi SK, Basit S, Ali N, Ansar M, Ahmad W. Novel mutations in the keratin-74 (KRT74) gene underlie autosomal dominant woolly hair/hypotrichosis in Pakistani families. Hum Genet. 2011;129(4): 419-24.

[24] Fujimoto A, Farooq M, Fujikawa H, Inoue A, Ohyama M, Ehama R, Nakanishi J, Hagihara M, Iwabuchi T, Aoki J, Ito M, Shimomura Y. A Missense Mutation within the Helix Initiation Motif of the Keratin K71 Gene Underlies Autosomal Dominant Woolly Hair/Hypotrichosis. J Invest Dermatol. 2012;132(10): 2342-9. doi: 10.1038/jid.2012.154.

[25] Langbein L, Rogers MA, Praetzel S, Winter H, Schweizer J. K6irs1, K6irs2, K6irs3, and K6irs4 represent the inner-root-sheath-specific type II epithelial keratins of the human hair follicle. J Invest Dermatol. 2003;120(4): 512-22.

[26] Kikkawa Y, Oyama A, Ishii R, Miura I, Amano T, Ishii Y, Yoshikawa Y, Masuya H, Wakana S, Shiroishi T, Taya C, Yonekawa H. A small deletion hotspot in the type II keratin gene mK6irs1/Krt2-6g on mouse chromosome 15, a candidate for causing the wavy hair of the caracul (Ca) mutation. Genetics. 2003;165(2): 721-33.

[27] Peters T, Sedlmeier R, Büssow H, Runkel F, Lüers GH, Korthaus D, Fuchs H, Hrabé de Angelis M, Stumm G, Russ AP, Porter RM, Augustin M, Franz T. Alopecia in a novel mouse model RCO3 is caused by mK6irs1 deficiency. J Invest Dermatol. 2003;121(4): 674-80.

[28] Kuramoto T, Hirano R, Kuwamura M, Serikawa T. Identification of the rat Rex mutation as a 7-bp deletion at splicing acceptor site of the Krt71 gene. J Vet Med Sci. 2010;72(7): 909-12.

[29] Gandolfi B, Outerbridge CA, Beresford LG, Myers JA, Pimentel M, Alhaddad H, Grahn JC, Grahn RA, Lyons LA. The naked truth: Sphynx and Devon Rex cat breed mutations in KRT71. Mamm Genome. 2010;21(9-10): 509-15.

[30] Cadieu E, Neff MW, Quignon P, Walsh K, Chase K, Parker HG, Vonholdt BM, Rhue A, Boyko A, Byers A, Wong A, Mosher DS, Elkahloun AG, Spady TC, André C, Lark KG, Cargill M, Bustamante CD, Wayne RK, Ostrander EA. Coat variation in the domestic dog is governed by variants in three genes. Science. 2009;326(5949): 150-3.

[31] McGrath JA. Inherited disorders of desmosomes. Australas J Dermatol. 2005;46(4): 221-9.

[32] Kljuic A, Bazzi H, Sundberg JP, Martinez-Mir A, O'Shaughnessy R, Mahoney MG, Levy M, Montagutelli X, Ahmad W, Aita VM, Gordon D, Uitto J, Whiting D, Ott J, Fischer S, Gilliam TC, Jahoda CA, Morris RJ, Panteleyev AA, Nguyen VT, Christiano AM. Desmoglein 4 in hair follicle differentiation and epidermal adhesion: evidence from inherited hypotrichosis and acquired pemphigus vulgaris. Cell. 2003;113(2): 249-60.

[33] Shimomura Y, Sakamoto F, Kariya N, Matsunaga K, Ito M. Mutations in the desmoglein 4 gene are associated with monilethrix-like congenital hypotrichosis. J Invest Dermatol. 2006;126(6):1281-5.

[34] Schaffer JV, Bazzi H, Vitebsky A, Witkiewicz A, Kovich OI, Kamino H, Shapiro LS, Amin SP, Orlow SJ, Christiano AM. Mutations in the desmoglein 4 gene underlie localized autosomal recessive hypotrichosis with monilethrix hairs and congenital scalp erosions. J Invest Dermatol. 2006;126(6): 1286-91.

[35] Zlotogorski A, Marek D, Horev L, Abu A, Ben-Amitai D, Gerad L, Ingber A, Frydman M, Reznik-Wolf H, Vardy DA, Pras E. An autosomal recessive form of monilethrix is caused by mutations in DSG4: clinical overlap with localized autosomal recessive hypotrichosis. J Invest Dermatol. 2006;126(6): 1292-6.

[36] Bazzi H, Getz A, Mahoney MG, Ishida-Yamamoto A, Langbein L, Wahl JK 3rd, Christiano AM. Desmoglein 4 is expressed in highly differentiated keratinocytes and trichocytes in human epidermis and hair follicle. Differentiation. 2006;74(2-3): 129-40.

[37] Ayub M, Basit S, Jelani M, Ur Rehman F, Iqbal M, Yasinzai M, Ahmad W. A homozygous nonsense mutation in the human desmocollin-3 (DSC3) gene underlies hereditary hypotrichosis and recurrent skin vesicles. Am J Hum Genet. 2009;85(4): 515-20.

[38] Payne AS. No evidence of skin blisters with human desmocollin-3 gene mutation. Am J Hum Genet. 2010;86(2): 292.

[39] McKoy G, Protonotarios N, Crosby A, Tsatsopoulou A, Anastasakis A, Coonar A, Norman M, Baboonian C, Jeffery S, McKenna WJ. Identification of a deletion in plakoglobin in arrhythmogenic right ventricular cardiomyopathy with palmoplantar keratoderma and woolly hair (Naxos disease). Lancet. 2000;355(9221): 2119-24.

[40] Norgett EE, Hatsell SJ, Carvajal-Huerta L, Cabezas JC, Common J, Purkis PE, Whittock N, Leigh IM, Stevens HP, Kelsell DP. Recessive mutation in desmoplakin disrupts desmoplakin-intermediate filament interactions and causes dilated cardiomyopathy, woolly hair and keratoderma. Hum Mol Genet. 2000;9(18): 2761-6.

[41] McGrath JA, McMillan JR, Shemanko CS, Runswick SK, Leigh IM, Lane EB, Garrod DR, Eady RA. Mutations in the plakophilin 1 gene result in ectodermal dysplasia/skin fragility syndrome. Nat Genet. 1997;17(2): 240-4.

[42] Ishida-Yamamoto A, Igawa S, Kishibe M. Order and disorder in corneocyte adhesion. J Dermatol. 2011;38(7): 645-54. doi: 10.1111/j.1346-8138.2011.01227.x.

[43] Mils V, Vincent C, Croute F, Serre G. The expression of desmosomal and corneodesmosomal antigens shows specific variations during the terminal differentiation of epidermis and hair follicle epithelia. J Histochem Cytochem. 1992;40(9): 1329-37.

[44] Levy-Nissenbaum E, Betz RC, Frydman M, Simon M, Lahat H, Bakhan T, Goldman B, Bygum A, Pierick M, Hillmer AM, Jonca N, Toribio J, Kruse R, Dewald G, Cichon S, Kubisch C, Guerrin M, Serre G, Nöthen MM, Pras E. Hypotrichosis simplex of the scalp is associated with nonsense mutations in CDSN encoding corneodesmosin. Nat Genet. 2003;34(2): 151-3.

[45] Caubet C, Bousset L, Clemmensen O, Sourigues Y, Bygum A, Chavanas S, Coudane F, Hsu CY, Betz RC, Melki R, Simon M, Serre G. A new amyloidosis caused by fibrillar aggregates of mutated corneodesmosin. FASEB J. 2010;24(9): 3416-26.

[46] Chavanas S, Bodemer C, Rochat A, Hamel-Teillac D, Ali M, Irvine AD, Bonafé JL, Wilkinson J, Taïeb A, Barrandon Y, Harper JI, de Prost Y, Hovnanian A. Mutations in SPINK5, encoding a serine protease inhibitor, cause Netherton syndrome. Nat Genet. 2000;25(2): 141-2.

[47] Komatsu N, Takata M, Otsuki N, Ohka R, Amano O, Takehara K, Saijoh K. Elevated stratum corneum hydrolytic activity in Netherton syndrome suggests an inhibitory

regulation of desquamation by SPINK5-derived peptides. J Invest Dermatol. 2002;118(3): 436-43.

[48] Yang T, Liang D, Koch PJ, Hohl D, Kheradmand F, Overbeek PA. Epidermal detachment, desmosomal dissociation, and destabilization of corneodesmosin in Spink5-/- mice. Genes Dev. 2004;18(19): 2354-8.

[49] Basel-Vanagaite L, Attia R, Ishida-Yamamoto A, Rainshtein L, Ben Amitai D, Lurie R, Pasmanik-Chor M, Indelman M, Zvulunov A, Saban S, Magal N, Sprecher E, Shohat M. Autosomal recessive ichthyosis with hypotrichosis caused by a mutation in ST14, encoding type II transmembrane serine protease matriptase. Am J Hum Genet. 2007;80(3): 467-77.

[50] Jamora C, DasGupta R, Kocieniewski P, Fuchs E. Links between signal transduction, transcription and adhesion in epithelial bud development. Nature. 2003;422(6929): 317-22.

[51] Samuelov L, Sprecher E, Tsuruta D, Bíró T, Kloepper JE, Paus R. P-Cadherin Regulates Human Hair Growth and Cycling via Canonical Wnt Signaling and Transforming Growth Factor-β2. J Invest Dermatol. 2012;132(10): 2332-41. doi: 10.1038/jid.2012.171.

[52] Sprecher E, Bergman R, Richard G, Lurie R, Shalev S, Petronius D, Shalata A, Anbinder Y, Leibu R, Perlman I, Cohen N, Szargel R. Hypotrichosis with juvenile macular dystrophy is caused by a mutation in CDH3, encoding P-cadherin. Nat Genet. 2001;29(2): 134-6.

[53] Kjaer KW, Hansen L, Schwabe GC, Marques-de-Faria AP, Eiberg H, Mundlos S, Tommerup N, Rosenberg T. Distinct CDH3 mutations cause ectodermal dysplasia, ectrodactyly, macular dystrophy (EEM syndrome). J Med Genet. 2005;42(4): 292-8.

[54] Indelman M, Hamel CP, Bergman R, Nischal KK, Thompson D, Surget MO, Ramon M, Ganthos H, Miller B, Richard G, Lurie R, Leibu R, Russell-Eggitt I, Sprecher E. Phenotypic diversity and mutation spectrum in hypotrichosis with juvenile macular dystrophy. J Invest Dermatol. 2003;121(5): 1217-20.

[55] Richard G. Connexins: a connection with the skin. Exp Dermatol. 2000;9(2): 77-96.

[56] Lamartine J, Munhoz Essenfelder G, Kibar Z, Lanneluc I, Callouet E, Laoudj D, Lemaître G, Hand C, Hayflick SJ, Zonana J, Antonarakis S, Radhakrishna U, Kelsell DP, Christianson AL, Pitaval A, Der Kaloustian V, Fraser C, Blanchet-Bardon C, Rouleau GA, Waksman G. Mutations in GJB6 cause hidrotic ectodermal dysplasia. Nat Genet. 2000;26(2): 142-4.

[57] Richard G, Rouan F, Willoughby CE, Brown N, Chung P, Ryynänen M, Jabs EW, Bale SJ, DiGiovanna JJ, Uitto J, Russell L. Missense mutations in GJB2 encoding connexin-26 cause the ectodermal dysplasia keratitis-ichthyosis-deafness syndrome. Am J Hum Genet. 2002;70(5): 1341-8.

[58] Jan AY, Amin S, Ratajczak P, Richard G, Sybert VP. Genetic heterogeneity of KID syndrome: identification of a Cx30 gene (GJB6) mutation in a patient with KID syndrome and congenital atrichia. J Invest Dermatol. 2004;122(5): 1108-13.

[59] Salomon D, Masgrau E, Vischer S, Ullrich S, Dupont E, Sappino P, Saurat JH, Meda P. Topography of mammalian connexins in human skin. J Invest Dermatol. 1994;103(2): 240-7.

[60] Essenfelder GM, Larderet G, Waksman G, Lamartine J. Gene structure and promoter analysis of the human GJB6 gene encoding connexin 30. Gene. 2005;350(1): 33-40.

[61] Brandner JM, McIntyre M, Kief S, Wladykowski E, Moll I. Expression and localization of tight junction-associated proteins in human hair follicles. Arch Dermatol Res. 2003;295(5): 211-21.

[62] Hadj-Rabia S, Baala L, Vabres P, Hamel-Teillac D, Jacquemin E, Fabre M, Lyonnet S, De Prost Y, Munnich A, Hadchouel M, Smahi A. Claudin-1 gene mutations in neonatal sclerosing cholangitis associated with ichthyosis: a tight junction disease. Gastroenterology. 2004;127(5): 1386-90.

[63] Celli J, Duijf P, Hamel BC, Bamshad M, Kramer B, Smits AP, Newbury-Ecob R, Hennekam RC, Van Buggenhout G, van Haeringen A, Woods CG, van Essen AJ, de Waal R, Vriend G, Haber DA, Yang A, McKeon F, Brunner HG, van Bokhoven H. Heterozygous germline mutations in the p53 homolog p63 are the cause of EEC syndrome. Cell. 1999;99(2): 143-53.

[64] McGrath JA, Duijf PH, Doetsch V, Irvine AD, de Waal R, Vanmolkot KR, Wessagowit V, Kelly A, Atherton DJ, Griffiths WA, Orlow SJ, van Haeringen A, Ausems MG, Yang A, McKeon F, Bamshad MA, Brunner HG, Hamel BC, van Bokhoven H. Hay-Wells syndrome is caused by heterozygous missense mutations in the SAM domain of p63. Hum Mol Genet. 2001;10(3): 221-9.

[65] Kantaputra PN, Hamada T, Kumchai T, McGrath JA. Heterozygous mutation in the SAM domain of p63 underlies Rapp-Hodgkin ectodermal dysplasia. J Dent Res. 2003;82(6): 433-7.

[66] Shimomura Y, Wajid M, Shapiro L, Christiano AM. P-cadherin is a p63 target gene with a crucial role in the developing human limb bud and hair follicle. Development. 2008;135(4): 743-53.

[67] Schlake T, Schorpp M, Maul-Pavicic A, Malashenko AM, Boehm T. Forkhead/winged-helix transcription factor Whn regulates hair keratin gene expression: molecular analysis of the nude skin phenotype. Dev Dyn. 2000;217(4): 368-76.

[68] Frank J, Pignata C, Panteleyev AA, Prowse DM, Baden H, Weiner L, Gaetaniello L, Ahmad W, Pozzi N, Cserhalmi-Friedman PB, Aita VM, Uyttendaele H, Gordon D, Ott J, Brissette JL, Christiano AM. Exposing the human nude phenotype. Nature. 1999;398(6727): 473-4.

[69] Panteleyev AA, Botchkareva NV, Sundberg JP, Christiano AM, Paus R. The role of the hairless (hr) gene in the regulation of hair follicle catagen transformation. Am J Pathol. 1999;155(1): 159-71.

[70] Ahmad W, Faiyaz ul Haque M, Brancolini V, Tsou HC, ul Haque S, Lam H, Aita VM, Owen J, deBlaquiere M, Frank J, Cserhalmi-Friedman PB, Leask A, McGrath JA,

Peacocke M, Ahmad M, Ott J, Christiano AM. Alopecia universalis associated with a mutation in the human hairless gene. Science. 1998;279(5351): 720-4.

[71] Sprecher E, Bergman R, Szargel R, Friedman-Birnbaum R, Cohen N. Identification of a genetic defect in the hairless gene in atrichia with papular lesions: evidence for phenotypic heterogeneity among inherited atrichias. Am J Hum Genet. 1999;64(5): 1323-9.

[72] van Steensel M, Smith FJ, Steijlen PM, Kluijt I, Stevens HP, Messenger A, Kremer H, Dunnill MG, Kennedy C, Munro CS, Doherty VR, McGrath JA, Covello SP, Coleman CM, Uitto J, McLean WH. The gene for hypotrichosis of Marie Unna maps between D8S258 and D8S298: exclusion of the hr gene by cDNA and genomic sequencing. Am J Hum Genet. 1999;65(2): 413-9.

[73] Wen Y, Liu Y, Xu Y, Zhao Y, Hua R, Wang K, Sun M, Li Y, Yang S, Zhang XJ, Kruse R, Cichon S, Betz RC, Nöthen MM, van Steensel MA, van Geel M, Steijlen PM, Hohl D, Huber M, Dunnill GS, Kennedy C, Messenger A, Munro CS, Terrinoni A, Hovnanian A, Bodemer C, de Prost Y, Paller AS, Irvine AD, Sinclair R, Green J, Shang D, Liu Q, Luo Y, Jiang L, Chen HD, Lo WH, McLean WH, He CD, Zhang X. Loss-of-function mutations of an inhibitory upstream ORF in the human hairless transcript cause Marie Unna hereditary hypotrichosis. Nat Genet. 2009;41(2): 228-33.

[74] Fantauzzo KA, Bazzi H, Jahoda CA, Christiano AM. Dynamic expression of the zinc-finger transcription factor Trps1 during hair follicle morphogenesis and cycling. Gene Expr Patterns. 2008;8(2): 51-7.

[75] Fantauzzo KA, Christiano AM. Trps1 activates a network of secreted Wnt inhibitors and transcription factors crucial to vibrissa follicle morphogenesis. Development. 2012;139(1): 203-14.

[76] Momeni P, Glöckner G, Schmidt O, von Holtum D, Albrecht B, Gillessen-Kaesbach G, Hennekam R, Meinecke P, Zabel B, Rosenthal A, Horsthemke B, Lüdecke HJ. Mutations in a new gene, encoding a zinc-finger protein, cause tricho-rhino-phalangeal syndrome type I. Nat Genet. 2000;24(1): 71-4.

[77] Lüdecke HJ, Schaper J, Meinecke P, Momeni P, Gross S, von Holtum D, Hirche H, Abramowicz MJ, Albrecht B, Apacik C, Christen HJ, Claussen U, Devriendt K, Fastnacht E, Forderer A, Friedrich U, Goodship TH, Greiwe M, Hamm H, Hennekam RC, Hinkel GK, Hoeltzenbein M, Kayserili H, Majewski F, Mathieu M, McLeod R, Midro AT, Moog U, Nagai T, Niikawa N, Orstavik KH, Plöchl E, Seitz C, Schmidtke J, Tranebjaerg L, Tsukahara M, Wittwer B, Zabel B, Gillessen-Kaesbach G, Horsthemke B. Genotypic and phenotypic spectrum in tricho-rhino-phalangeal syndrome types I and III. Am J Hum Genet. 2001;68(1): 81-91.

[78] Irrthum A, Devriendt K, Chitayat D, Matthijs G, Glade C, Steijlen PM, Fryns JP, Van Steensel MA, Vikkula M. Mutations in the transcription factor gene SOX18 underlie recessive and dominant forms of hypotrichosis-lymphedema-telangiectasia. Am J Hum Genet. 2003;72(6): 1470-8

[79] Price JA, Bowden DW, Wright JT, Pettenati MJ, Hart TC. Identification of a mutation in DLX3 associated with tricho-dento-osseous (TDO) syndrome. Hum Mol Genet. 1998;7(3): 563-9.

[80] Kere J, Srivastava AK, Montonen O, Zonana J, Thomas N, Ferguson B, Munoz F, Morgan D, Clarke A, Baybayan P, Chen EY, Ezer S, Saarialho-Kere U, de la Chapelle A, Schlessinger D. X-linked anhidrotic (hypohidrotic) ectodermal dysplasia is caused by mutation in a novel transmembrane protein. Nat Genet. 1996;13(4): 409-16.

[81] Monreal AW, Ferguson BM, Headon DJ, Street SL, Overbeek PA, Zonana J. Mutations in the human homologue of mouse dl cause autosomal recessive and dominant hypohidrotic ectodermal dysplasia. Nat Genet. 1999;22(4): 366-9.

[82] Headon DJ, Emmal SA, Ferguson BM, Tucker AS, Justice MJ, Sharpe PT, Zonana J, Overbeek PA. Gene defect in ectodermal dysplasia implicates a death domain adapter in development. Nature. 2001;414(6866): 913-6.

[83] Bayés M, Hartung AJ, Ezer S, Pispa J, Thesleff I, Srivastava AK, Kere J. The anhidrotic ectodermal dysplasia gene (EDA) undergoes alternative splicing and encodes ectodysplasin-A with deletion mutations in collagenous repeats. Hum Mol Genet. 1998;7(11): 1661-9.

[84] Yan M, Wang LC, Hymowitz SG, Schilbach S, Lee J, Goddard A, de Vos AM, Gao WQ, Dixit VM. Two-amino acid molecular switch in an epithelial morphogen that regulates binding to two distinct receptors. Science. 2000;290(5491): 523-7.

[85] Mikkola ML. Molecular aspects of hypohidrotic ectodermal dysplasia. Am J Med Genet A. 2009;149A(9): 2031-6.

[86] Wisniewski SA, Trzeciak WH. A rare heterozygous TRAF6 variant is associated with hypohidrotic ectodermal dysplasia. Br J Dermatol. 2012;166(6):1353-6. doi: 10.1111/j.1365-2133.2012.10871.x.

[87] Adaimy L, Chouery E, Megarbane H, Mroueh S, Delague V, Nicolas E, Belguith H, de Mazancourt P, Megarbane A. Mutation in WNT10A is associated with an autosomal recessive ectodermal dysplasia: the odonto-onycho-dermal dysplasia. Am J Hum Genet. 2007;81(4): 821-8.

[88] Cluzeau C, Hadj-Rabia S, Jambou M, Mansour S, Guigue P, Masmoudi S, Bal E, Chassaing N, Vincent MC, Viot G, Clauss F, Manière MC, Toupenay S, Le Merrer M, Lyonnet S, Cormier-Daire V, Amiel J, Faivre L, de Prost Y, Munnich A, Bonnefont JP, Bodemer C, Smahi A. Only four genes (EDA1, EDAR, EDARADD, and WNT10A) account for 90% of hypohidrotic/anhidrotic ectodermal dysplasia cases. Hum Mutat. 2011;32(1): 70-2.

[89] Zhang Y, Tomann P, Andl T, Gallant NM, Huelsken J, Jerchow B, Birchmeier W, Paus R, Piccolo S, Mikkola ML, Morrisey EE, Overbeek PA, Scheidereit C, Millar SE, Schmidt-Ullrich R. Reciprocal requirements for EDA/EDAR/NF-kappaB and Wnt/beta-catenin signaling pathways in hair follicle induction. Dev Cell. 2009;17(1): 49-61.

[90] Baumer A, Belli S, Trüeb RM, Schinzel A. An autosomal dominant form of hereditary hypotrichosis simplex maps to 18p11.32-p11.23 in an Italian family. Eur J Hum Genet. 2000;8(6): 443-8.

[91] Shimomura Y, Agalliu D, Vonica A, Luria V, Wajid M, Baumer A, Belli S, Petukhova L, Schinzel A, Brivanlou AH, Barres BA, Christiano AM. APCDD1 is a novel Wnt inhibitor mutated in hereditary hypotrichosis simplex. Nature. 2010;464(7291): 1043-7.

[92] Li M, Cheng R, Zhuang Y, Yao Z. A recurrent mutation in the APCDD1 gene responsible for hereditary hypotrichosis simplex in a large Chinese family. Br J Dermatol. 2012. doi: 10.1111/j.1365-2133.2012.11001.x.

[93] Takahashi T, Kamimura A, Hamazono-Matsuoka T, Honda S. Phosphatidic acid has a potential to promote hair growth in vitro and in vivo, and activates mitogen-activated protein kinase/extracellular signal-regulated kinase kinase in hair epithelial cells. J Invest Dermatol. 2003;121(3): 448-56.

[94] Kazantseva A, Goltsov A, Zinchenko R, Grigorenko AP, Abrukova AV, Moliaka YK, Kirillov AG, Guo Z, Lyle S, Ginter EK, Rogaev EI. Human hair growth deficiency is linked to a genetic defect in the phospholipase gene LIPH. Science. 2006;314(5801): 982-5.

[95] Shimomura Y, Wajid M, Petukhova L, Shapiro L, Christiano AM. Mutations in the lipase H gene underlie autosomal recessive woolly hair/hypotrichosis. J Invest Dermatol. 2009;129(3): 622-8.

[96] Shimomura Y. Congenital hair loss disorders: rare, but not too rare. J Dermatol. 2012;39(1): 3-10. doi: 10.1111/j.1346-8138.2011.01395.x.

[97] Sonoda H, Aoki J, Hiramatsu T, Ishida M, Bandoh K, Nagai Y, Taguchi R, Inoue K, Arai H. A novel phosphatidic acid-selective phospholipase A1 that produces lysophosphatidic acid. J Biol Chem. 2002;277(37): 34254-63.

[98] Pasternack SM, von Kügelgen I, Al Aboud K, Lee YA, Rüschendorf F, Voss K, Hillmer AM, Molderings GJ, Franz T, Ramirez A, Nürnberg P, Nöthen MM, Betz RC. G protein-coupled receptor P2Y5 and its ligand LPA are involved in maintenance of human hair growth. Nat Genet. 2008;40(3): 329-34.

[99] Shimomura Y, Wajid M, Ishii Y, Shapiro L, Petukhova L, Gordon D, Christiano AM. Disruption of P2RY5, an orphan G protein-coupled receptor, underlies autosomal recessive woolly hair. Nat Genet. 2008;40(3): 335-9.

[100] Yanagida K, Masago K, Nakanishi H, Kihara Y, Hamano F, Tajima Y, Taguchi R, Shimizu T, Ishii S. Identification and characterization of a novel lysophosphatidic acid receptor, p2y5/LPA6. J Biol Chem. 2009;284(26): 17731-41.

[101] Inoue A, Arima N, Ishiguro J, Prestwich GD, Arai H, Aoki J. LPA-producing enzyme PA-PLA$_{1}\alpha$ regulates hair follicle development by modulating EGFR signalling. EMBO J. 2011;30(20): 4248-60. doi: 10.1038/emboj.2011.296.

[102] Blaydon DC, Biancheri P, Di WL, Plagnol V, Cabral RM, Brooke MA, van Heel DA, Ruschendorf F, Toynbee M, Walne A, O'Toole EA, Martin JE, Lindley K, Vulliamy T,

Abrams DJ, MacDonald TT, Harper JI, Kelsell DP. Inflammatory skin and bowel disease linked to ADAM17 deletion. N Engl J Med. 2011;365(16): 1502-8.

[103] Wheeler DA, Srinivasan M, Egholm M, Shen Y, Chen L, McGuire A, He W, Chen YJ, Makhijani V, Roth GT, Gomes X, Tartaro K, Niazi F, Turcotte CL, Irzyk GP, Lupski JR, Chinault C, Song XZ, Liu Y, Yuan Y, Nazareth L, Qin X, Muzny DM, Margulies M, Weinstock GM, Gibbs RA, Rothberg JM. The complete genome of an individual by massively parallel DNA sequencing. Nature. 2008;452(7189): 872-6.

Chapter 2

Epidermolysis Bullosa Simplex

Ken Natsuga

Additional information is available at the end of the chapter

http://dx.doi.org/10.5772/54609

1. Introduction

Epidermolysis bullosa (EB) is a heterogeneous group of congenital disorders characterized by skin blister formation. EB is subdivided into three main subtypes (EB simplex (EBS), junctional EB (JEB) and dystrophic EB (DEB)) and one minor subtype (Kindler syndrome (KS)), according to the level of skin split [1].

The EBS subtype can be defined as EBS with blisters within epidermal basal keratinocytes or above, and it is distinguished from other subtypes whose levels of blister formation are deeper (JEB and DEB) or variable (KS). Mutations in several genes have been identified as being responsible for EBS phenotypes. The clinical manifestations of EBS vary greatly depending on the causative genes. Some EBS subtypes are mild and tend to improve with age, whereas others are severe and often associated with early demise and/or other organ involvement. This chapter introduces the clinical and histological characteristics and classifications of EBS. Subsequently, each protein that is defective in EBS is discussed, as are animal models of the disease.

2. Overview of epidermolysis bullosa simplex

Mutations in genes encoding keratinocyte components involved in the organization of the cytoskeleton or cell-cell junctions are responsible for EBS. EBS can be subclassified into basal and suprabasal according to the level of skin split [1, 2] **(Table 1)**.

Basal EBS is caused by defects in skin basement membrane (BMZ) proteins. **Figure 1** diagrams the skin BMZ. Among the BMZ components, keratin 5/14 and plectin are the main targets in EBS [3, 4]. A few EBS cases have been reported to have mutations in *ITGB4* and *COL17*, which encode β4 integrin and type XVII collagen, respectively [5, 6]. Recently, BPAG1-e was added to the list of basal EBS target proteins [7, 8].

	Subtype	Target gene (protein)
EBS	Suprabasal EBS	*PKP1* (plakophilin-1)
		DSP (desmoplakin)
		JUP (plakoglobin)
	Basal EBS	*KRT5* (keratin 5)
		KRT14 (keratin 14)
		PLEC (plectin)
		COL17 (type XVII collagen)
		ITGB4 (β4 integrin)

Table 1. Classification of EBS [1, 2]

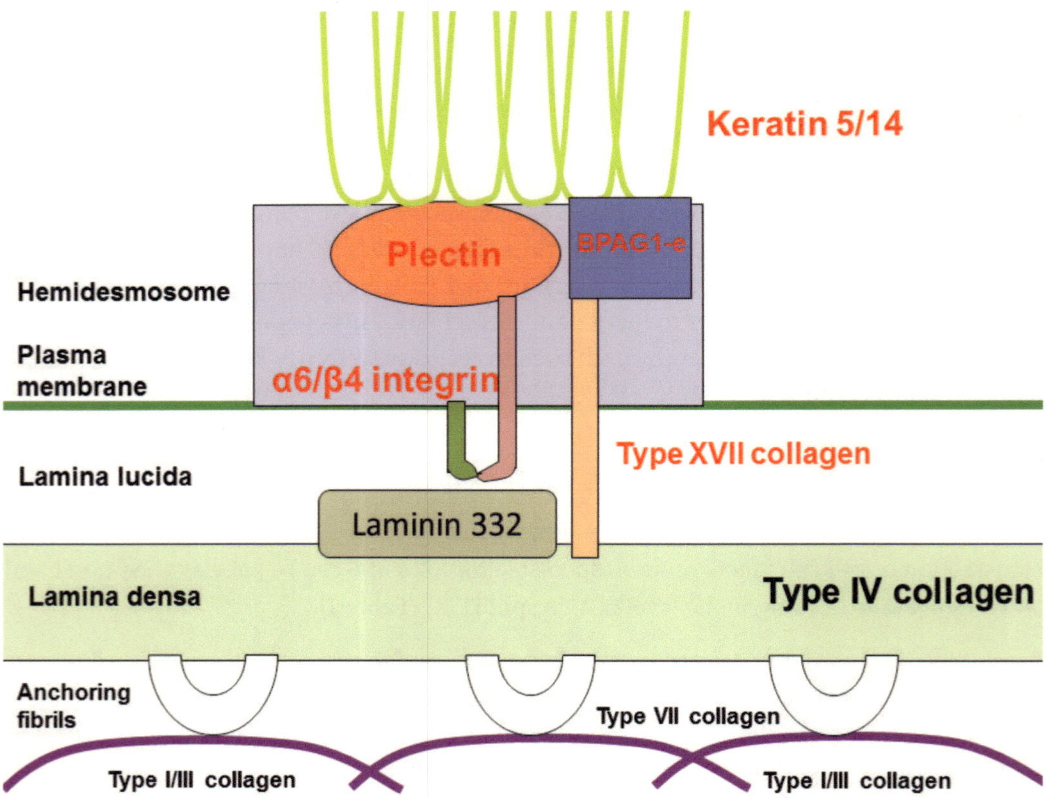

Figure 1. Schematic of the skin basement membrane zone. Components in red characters are target proteins of basal EBS.

In contrast, suprabasal EBS is associated with abnormalities in desmosomal proteins (**Figure 2**). So far, plakophilin-1, plakoglobin and desmoplakin are known to be the target proteins of suprabasal EBS [2, 9-11].

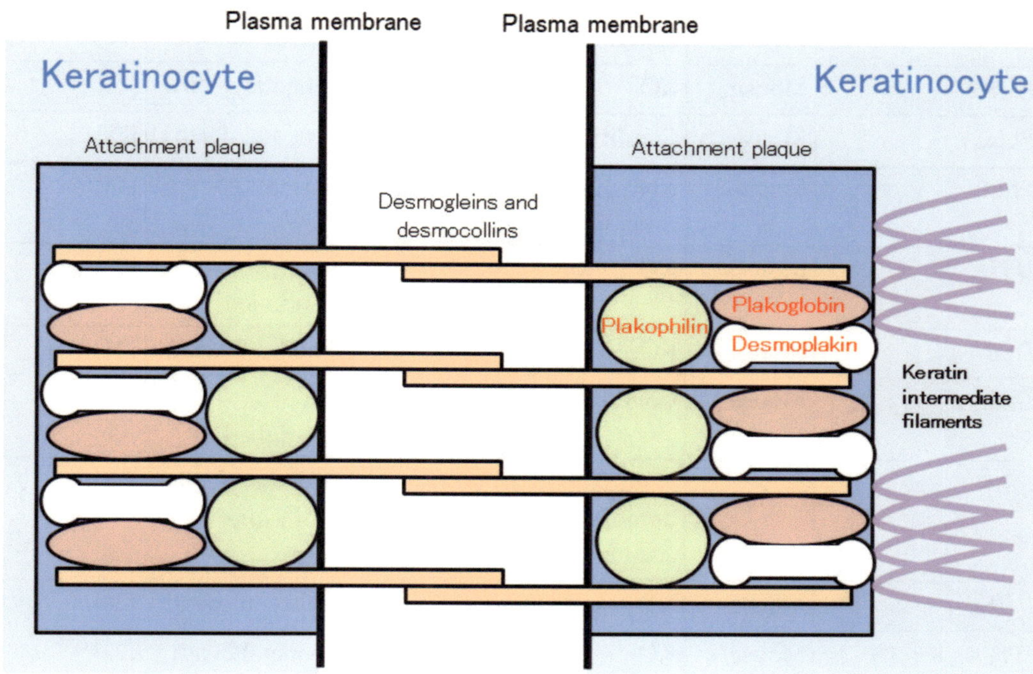

Figure 2. Schematic of desmosomes. Components in red characters are target proteins of suprabasal EBS.

Animal models have been used to clarify the function of some proteins and to develop new therapies for human diseases. Animal models of EB were reviewed recently [12, 13]. However, some new animal models have emerged since then [14, 15], and other transgenic mice with abnormalities in desmosomal proteins should be added to the list of EB animal models because of the introduction of the concept of "suprabasal EBS" [1]. **Table 2** summarizes animal models of EBS.

Causative Gene	Species	Type	Survival	Reference
KRT5	Mouse	KO	Neonatal death	[16]
KRT5	Cow	Naturally occurring (a heterozygous missense mutation)	Not mentioned	[17]
KRT14	Mouse	Tg (expressing truncated protein)	Neonatal death	[18]
KRT14	Mouse	KO	Neonatal death	[19]
KRT14	Mouse	KI	Neonatal death	[20]
KRT14	Mouse	KI (an inducible model)	Not mentioned	[20]
PLEC	Mouse	KO	Neonatal death	[21]
PLEC	Mouse	Conditional KO	Neonatal death	[22]
PLEC	Mouse	KI (expressing EBS-Ogna mutation)	Normal	[14]
DST	Mouse	KO	Not mentioned	[23]
DSP	Mouse	KO	Embryonicdeath	[24]
DSP	Mouse	Conditional KO	Not mentioned	[25]
PKP1	Dog	Naturally occurring (a homozygous splice donor site mutation)	Neonatal death (6 of 9 affected dogs)	[15]
JUP	Mouse	KO	Embryonicdeath	[26]
ITGB4	Mouse	KO	Neonatal death	[27]
ITGB4	Mouse	KO	Neonatal death	[28]
ITGB4	Mouse	Partial ablation (expressing ectodomain of β4 integrin)	Neonatal death	[29]
ITGB4	Mouse	Conditional KO	Not mentioned	[30]
COL17A1	Mouse	KO	Prolonged survival in 20% of mice	[31]

KO: knockout; Tg: transgenic; KI: knock-in

Table 2. Animal models of EBS [12-15]

3. Target proteins in basal EBS

3.1. Keratin 5/14

Recent brilliant reviews have addressed keratins and EBS [3, 32]. Here we focus on the history, mutation analysis, animal models and future therapeutics of keratin-associated EBS from the physician's point of view.

Keratin is one of the most abundant components of the epithelial cytoskeleton [33]. Typically, type I and type II keratins form heteropolymers that function in cells [34]. Keratin 5 (K5) and keratin 14 (K14) are specifically expressed in epidermal basal cells [34, 35] (**Figure 1**). In the 1980's, disorganization of those keratins was recognized in the basal keratinocytes of EBS patients [36, 37]. From those findings, it had been hypothesized that EBS patients have mutations in *KRT5* or *KRT14*, which encodes K5 or K14, respectively. In the early 1990's, transgenic mice overexpressing mutated K14 were reported to have severe skin fragility [18]. Soon after this discovery, two groups of researchers identified EBS cases with heterozygosity for *KRT14* missense mutations [38, 39], which were followed by the identification of the first EBS family with a heterozygous *KRT5* mutation [40]. Since then, several hundreds of EBS patients have been described as having *KRT5* or *KRT14* mutations and have been summarized in the Human Intermediate Filament Database (http://www.interfil.org/) [41].

There are several subtypes of keratin-associated EBS, as described in **Table 3** [1]. Classical and common EBS subtypes, in which traits are autosomal-dominantly inherited, are Dowling-Meara type EBS (EBS-DM), non Dowling-Meara type (EBS-gen-non-DM) and localized type (EBS-loc), from the severest to the mildest. Ultrastructurally, basal keratinocytes of EBS-DM are characterized by keratin aggregates [42]. Hot spots of the mutations in *KRT5* or *KRT14* are located within the helix-boundary motifs of each keratin [41]. A missense mutation in one allele of those regions (which leads to an amino acid alteration) typically exerts a dominant-negative effect on keratin organization. The severity of the clinical manifestations among EBS-DM, EBS-gen-non-DM and EBS-loc is generally determined by the site of the mutations and the difference between the original and the mutated amino acids [32]. However, it is not always easy to predict the phenotype from the underlying mutations and, in some cases, two different amino acid substitutions at the same codon result in different clinical manifestations [43, 44]. As a single amino-acid alteration does not necessarily cause a pathological change, *in vitro* and *in silico* systems to validate mutational effects have been proposed where keratin organization is visualized in cells transfected with mutated or wild-type keratins [44, 45].

The pathogenesis of EBS development through keratin mutations has also been demonstrated in animal models (**Table 2**). Following the discovery of transgenic mice overexpressing mutated K14 described above [18], *Krt5*-null and *Krt14*-null mice were reported to have a skin fragility phenotype [16, 19], although the condition of those mice was different from that of most EBS patients, where altered amino acids yield dominant-negative effects. Instead, those *Krt5*-null and *Krt14*-null mice show the phenotype of autosomal recessive EBS (EBS-AR) whose K5 or K14 is null [32]. To reproduce dominant-negative effects of mutated keratins in human EBS (EBS-DM, EBS-gen-non-DM and EBS-loc), inducible knock-in EBS model mice were generated, in which a *Krt14* missense mutation equivalent to human EBS mutation was introduced [20]. This inducible EBS model recapitulates the skin fragility seen in human patients with autosomal dominant EBS. Furthermore, there is one naturally occurring bovine with a heterozygous *KRT5* mutation [17]. This Friesian-Jersey crossbred bull exhibits the EBS phenotype.

EBS, Dowling-Meara (EBS-DM)	Classical EBS
EBS, other generalized (EBS, gen-nonDM)	Classical EBS
EBS, localized (EBS-loc)	Classical EBS
EBS, autosomal recessive (EBS-AR)	
EBS with mottled pigmentation (EBS-MP)	
EBS, migratory circinate (EBS-Migr)	

Table 3. Keratin-associated EBS

Therapeutic interventions for EBS have been confined to palliative modalities. However, recent innovations in RNA interference have led to therapeutic strategies for dominant-negative disorders including keratin-associated EBS, where aberrant mutated keratin is knocked down while normal keratin synthesis on another allele is left intact [46]. This RNAi strategy is promising and will be further validated in clinical trials.

3.2. Plectin

A comprehensive review paper has addressed EBS and plectin [4], although there have been several advances in this field since then [14, 47-49].

Plectin is a cross-linking protein between the cytoskeleton and membranous proteins including hemidesmosomal components (**Figure 1**). Plectin has been known to have many transcript isoforms that differ from each other in N-terminal sequences at the protein level [50]. Among the many transcript isoforms, plectin 1a is the one that is mainly expressed in epidermal keratinocytes [51]. In addition to 5′ transcript complexity, plectin has a rodless splicing variant [52]. There are several EBS subtypes that are caused by plectin deficiencies (**Table 4**).

In the mid-1990′s, mutations in the gene encoding plectin (*PLEC*) were discovered in patients with EBS with muscular dystrophy (EBS-MD) [53, 54]. Since then, many *PLEC* mutations, mostly located in the region encoding the rod domain of plectin, have been reported in EBS-MD patients [4, 47, 55].

EBS with muscular dystrophy (EBS-MD)	Autosomal recessive
EBS with pyloric atresia (EBS-PA)	
EBS with muscular dystrophy and pyloric atresia (EBS-MD-PA)	
EBS, Ogna (EBS-Og) →	Autosomal dominant

Table 4. Plectin-associated EBS

In 2005, two groups independently reported a new EBS subtype with *PLEC* mutations: EBS with pyloric atresia (EBS-PA) [56, 57]. EB with pyloric atresia (PA) had been known in patients with *ITGA6* or *ITGB4* mutations [58, 59]. However, skin specimens from those patients with integrin mutations show skin-split at the level of the lamina lucida, leading to the diagnosis of junctional EB (JEB). In contrast, EBS-PA cases with *PLEC* mutations were characterized by skin-split within epidermal basal cells [56].

The reason *PLEC* mutations lead to two distinct subtypes of EBS was clarified only recently. The development of monoclonal antibodies against several portions of plectin allowed us to understand the plectin expression patterns that distinguish between EBS-MD and EBS-PA [47]. EBS-MD skin typically shows the expression of rodless plectin without that of full-length plectin, whereas neither rodless nor full-length plectin is present in EBS-PA skin [47].

The next big question was whether EBS-MD and EBS-PA can occur simultaneously in a single patient or those two distinct EBS subtypes are mutually exclusive. Recently, one case was reported to have the phenotype of both EBS-MD and EBS-PA (EBS-MD-PA) [48]. The patient had truncation mutations at the last exon of *PLEC*, which resulted in the expression of diminished and shortened full-length and rodless plectin without the intermediate filament binding domain [48].

Apart from autosomal recessive EBS subtypes associated with *PLEC* mutations (EBS-MD, EBS-MD and EBS-MD-PA), there is one distinct autosomal dominant EBS with a *PLEC* mutation: EBS, Ogna (EBS-Og). EBS-Og is caused by a heterogeneous mutation of p. Arg2000Trp and is characterized by mild blister formation without MD or PA phenotype [4, 60]. To date, 5 unrelated families of EBS-Og have been reported to have the same mutation [49, 60].

Animal models of plectin-deficient EBS have been generated (**Table 2**). *Plec*-null mice show severe blistering phenotype and neonatal death [21], although gastrointestinal tracts were not investigated to confirm PA or PA-like lesions. Myofibril integrity is impaired in the skeletal and heart muscle of those mice [21]. Epidermis-specific ablation of plectin also elicits a severe blistering phenotype and early lethality in mice [22]. Furthermore, mice knocked-in with the murine equivalent mutation of EBS-Og show skin fragility due to epidermal-specific proteolysis of mutated plectin [14].

3.3. BPAG1-e

Dystonin, encoded by *DST*, has various isoforms in neural, muscle and epithelial tissue. BPAG1-e, also called BP230, is a major skin isoform of dystonin and a component of hemidesmosomes (**Figure 1**). BPAG1-e is known to be an autoantigen in bullous pemphigoid as well as type XVII collagen (C17) [61-63]. Since *COL17*, which encodes C17, was identified as a causative gene for non-Herlitz JEB [64], *DST*, which encodes BPAG1-e, had also been hypothesized for decades to be a target gene in other EB subtypes. However, it was only recently that mutations in *DST* were identified in autosomal recessive EBS patients [7, 8]. Those two patients typically had a mild acral blistering phenotype and had truncation mutations in the coiled-coil rod domain of BPAG1-e. Electron microscopy observation revealed loss of the inner plaque of hemidesmosomes in both cases [7, 8]. *Dst*-null mice show neural degeneration and mild skin fragility upon mechanical stress [23] (**Table 2**).

3.4. Miscellaneous

Mutations in *COL17* have been known to be responsible for non-Herlitz JEB (nH-JEB), in which the lamina lucida is the location of the skin-split as described above [64] (**Figure 1**). However, one case was reported to show a phenotype of EBS with *COL17* mutations [5]. The mutations found in that case caused a loss of intracellular C17 [5]. Furthermore, *Col17*-null mice were reported to show a reduced number of hypoplastic hemidesmosomal inner and outer attachment plaques with poor keratin filament attachment [31]. These findings suggest that *COL17* mutations can cause not only nH-JEB but also EBS, depending on the mutational sites.

$\alpha 6/\beta 4$ integrins are hemidesmosomal components that are encoded by *ITGA6/ITGB4*, respectively. (**Figure 1**). Those genes are also target genes in JEB (with or without PA), just as *COL17* is a target gene in nH-JEB. There is one autosomal recessive EBS case where the intracellular portion of $\beta 4$ integrin was deleted [6].

4. Target proteins in suprabasal EBS

4.1. Desmoplakin

Desmoplakin is a plakin family protein located in desmosome [55] (**Figure 2**). Two isoforms (desmoplakins I and II) are generated through alternative splicing [65]. Desmoplakin I is mainly expressed in the heart, whereas desmoplakin II is abundant in the skin [66]. In the early 1990's, desmoplakin was determined as a major autoantigen in paraneoplastic pemphigus [67, 68]. Mutations in the gene encoding desmoplakin, *DSP*, have been reported in several genodermatoses, mostly with cardiac manifestations [11, 69]. In 2005, a very severe EB case, referred to as lethal acantholytic epidermolysis bullosa (LAEB), was reported to have a homozygous deletion mutation in *DSP* [70]. The patient showed severe skin blistering and early demise. There have been only three reports on LAEB with *DSP* mutations [70-72]. Skin specimens in all the cases revealed acantholytic features in histopathology. From the correlation of clinical manifestations and mutational sites, it seems that complete or almost complete loss of desmoplakin might lead to LAEB [72]. However, at least one full-length desmoplakin (either isoform I or II) may be enough to prevent the development of LAEB [72].

There are two desmoplakin-associated EBS model animals (**Table 2**). The fact that *Dsp* knockout mice show embryonic lethality confirms that desmoplakin is essential in the early development of tissue architecture through embryogenesis [24]. Epidermis-specific ablation of *Dsp* elicits severe skin defects in newborn mice [25].

4.2. Plakophilin-1

Plakophilin-deficient EBS is listed in the newest classification of EB [1]. This entity has also been called ectodermal dysplasia-skin fragility syndrome (ED-SF). An excellent review on this EBS subtype was published recently [10]. The first case of ED-SF and the mutations in the gene encoding plakophilin-1, *PKP1*, were reported in 1997 [73]. Since then, many cases of ED-SF with *PKP1* mutations have been published. The clinical manifestations of ED-SF include skin fragility, perioral cracking, alopecia and palmoplantar keratoderma [10].

The desmosomal expression of plakophilin-1 (**Figure 2**) accounts for skin fragility and histological features of skin specimens characterized by widening of spaces between keratinocytes. However, the phenotype of ectodermal dysplasia may not be explained solely by desmosomal proteins. Recently, plakophilin-1 has been identified as a regulator of protein synthesis and proliferation through a pathway associated with eIF4A1 [74]. It is speculated that the role of plakophilin-1 in translation and proliferation is involved in abnormalities in skin appendages of ED-SF patients [74].

Mice models in which plakophilin-1 is defective have not been reported. However, there is a naturally occurring canine model with *PKP1* mutations that recapitulates human ED-SF [15] (**Table 2**). This family of Chesapeake Bay retriever dogs typically shows skin fragility and some ectodermal dysplasiac manifestations such as hair loss.

4.3. Plakoglobin

JUP, which encodes plakoglobin, was not listed as a causative gene of EB in the report of the Third International Consensus Meeting on Diagnosis and Classification of EB [1]. It was only recently that a homozygous nonsense mutation of this gene, leading to complete loss of plakoglobin, was revealed to be responsible for one subtype of suprabasal EBS [2]. Lethal congenital EB (LCEB), named by the authors, has manifestations similar to those of LAEB, which is caused by *DSP* mutations [2]. This similarity is accounted for by the expression pattern of plakoglobin and desmoplakin in desmosomes (**Figure 2**). This new entity is expected to be included in future classifications of EB [11].

Jup-null mice were reported much earlier than their human equivalents [26] (**Table 2**). Those mice show embryonic death with severe defects in the skin and heart [26].

5. Summary

Many genes are involved in the manifestations of EBS, as described in this chapter. The most common subtype is keratin-associated EBS caused by dominant-negative effects of aberrant mutated protein. RNAi strategies will be used in future clinical trials, although it is not easy to apply such therapies for all patients, because each patient has a different mutation. Tailor-made strategies will be required to correct each EBS mutation.

Other EBS subtypes are generally complicated with organ malfunction. The task of clinicians is to predict the prognosis of each EBS cases based on the causative genes. It is imperative to clarify what organs, other than the skin, will suffer dysfunction in each EBS case.

Author details

Ken Natsuga
Hokkaido University, Japan

6. References

[1] Fine JD, Eady RA, Bauer EA, Bauer JW, Bruckner-Tuderman L, Heagerty A, Hintner H, Hovnanian A, Jonkman MF, Leigh I, McGrath JA, Mellerio JE, Murrell DF, Shimizu H, Uitto J, Vahlquist A, Woodley D, Zambruno G. The classification of inherited epidermolysis bullosa (EB): Report of the Third International Consensus Meeting on Diagnosis and Classification of EB. J Am Acad Dermatol. 2008;58(6):931-950.

[2] Pigors M, Kiritsi D, Krumpelmann S, Wagner N, He Y, Podda M, Kohlhase J, Hausser I, Bruckner-Tuderman L, Has C. Lack of plakoglobin leads to lethal congenital epidermolysis bullosa: a novel clinico-genetic entity. Hum Mol Genet. 2011;20(9):1811-1819.

[3] Coulombe PA, Kerns ML, Fuchs E. Epidermolysis bullosa simplex: a paradigm for disorders of tissue fragility. J Clin Invest. 2009;119(7):1784-1793.

[4] Rezniczek GA, Walko G, Wiche G. Plectin gene defects lead to various forms of epidermolysis bullosa simplex. Dermatol Clin. 2010;28(1):33-41.

[5] Huber M, Floeth M, Borradori L, Schacke H, Rugg EL, Lane EB, Frenk E, Hohl D, Bruckner-Tuderman L. Deletion of the cytoplasmatic domain of BP180/collagen XVII causes a phenotype with predominant features of epidermolysis bullosa simplex. J Invest Dermatol. 2002;118(1):185-192.

[6] Jonkman MF, Pas HH, Nijenhuis M, Kloosterhuis G, Steege G. Deletion of a cytoplasmic domain of integrin beta4 causes epidermolysis bullosa simplex. J Invest Dermatol. 2002;119(6):1275-1281.

[7] Groves RW, Liu L, Dopping-Hepenstal PJ, Markus HS, Lovell PA, Ozoemena L, Lai-Cheong JE, Gawler J, Owaribe K, Hashimoto T, Mellerio JE, Mee JB, McGrath JA. A homozygous nonsense mutation within the dystonin gene coding for the coiled-coil

domain of the epithelial isoform of BPAG1 underlies a new subtype of autosomal recessive epidermolysis bullosa simplex. J Invest Dermatol. 2010;130(6):1551-1557.

[8] Liu L, Dopping-Hepenstal PJ, Lovell PA, Michael M, Horn H, Fong K, Lai-Cheong JE, Mellerio JE, Parsons M, McGrath JA. Autosomal recessive epidermolysis bullosa simplex due to loss of BPAG1-e expression. J Invest Dermatol. 2012;132(3 Pt 1):742-744.

[9] McGrath JA, Bolling MC, Jonkman MF. Lethal acantholytic epidermolysis bullosa. Dermatol Clin. 2010;28(1):131-135.

[10] McGrath JA, Mellerio JE. Ectodermal dysplasia-skin fragility syndrome. Dermatol Clin. 2010;28(1):125-129.

[11] Petrof G, Mellerio JE, McGrath JA. Desmosomal genodermatoses. Br J Dermatol. 2012;166(1):36-45.

[12] Bruckner-Tuderman L, McGrath JA, Robinson EC, Uitto J. Animal models of epidermolysis bullosa: update 2010. J Invest Dermatol. 2010;130(6):1485-1488.

[13] Natsuga K, Shinkuma S, Nishie W, Shimizu H. Animal models of epidermolysis bullosa. Dermatol Clin. 2010;28(1):137-142.

[14] Walko G, Vukasinovic N, Gross K, Fischer I, Sibitz S, Fuchs P, Reipert S, Jungwirth U, Berger W, Salzer U, Carugo O, Castanon MJ, Wiche G. Targeted proteolysis of plectin isoform 1a accounts for hemidesmosome dysfunction in mice mimicking the dominant skin blistering disease EBS-Ogna. PLoS Genet. 2011;7(12):e1002396.

[15] Olivry T, Linder KE, Wang P, Bizikova P, Bernstein JA, Dunston SM, Paps JS, Casal ML. Deficient plakophilin-1 expression due to a mutation in PKP1 causes ectodermal dysplasia-skin fragility syndrome in Chesapeake Bay retriever dogs. PLoS One. 2012;7(2):e32072.

[16] Peters B, Kirfel J, Bussow H, Vidal M, Magin TM. Complete cytolysis and neonatal lethality in keratin 5 knockout mice reveal its fundamental role in skin integrity and in epidermolysis bullosa simplex. Mol Biol Cell. 2001;12(6):1775-1789.

[17] Ford CA, Stanfield AM, Spelman RJ, Smits B, Ankersmidt-Udy AE, Cottier K, Holloway H, Walden A, Al-Wahb M, Bohm E, Snell RG, Sutherland GT. A mutation in bovine keratin 5 causing epidermolysis bullosa simplex, transmitted by a mosaic sire. J Invest Dermatol. 2005;124(6):1170-1176.

[18] Vassar R, Coulombe PA, Degenstein L, Albers K, Fuchs E. Mutant keratin expression in transgenic mice causes marked abnormalities resembling a human genetic skin disease. Cell. 1991;64(2):365-380.

[19] Lloyd C, Yu QC, Cheng J, Turksen K, Degenstein L, Hutton E, Fuchs E. The basal keratin network of stratified squamous epithelia: defining K15 function in the absence of K14. J Cell Biol. 1995;129(5):1329-1344.

[20] Cao T, Longley MA, Wang XJ, Roop DR. An inducible mouse model for epidermolysis bullosa simplex: implications for gene therapy. J Cell Biol. 2001;152(3):651-656.

[21] Andra K, Lassmann H, Bittner R, Shorny S, Fassler R, Propst F, Wiche G. Targeted inactivation of plectin reveals essential function in maintaining the integrity of skin, muscle, and heart cytoarchitecture. Genes Dev. 1997;11(23):3143-3156.

[22] Ackerl R, Walko G, Fuchs P, Fischer I, Schmuth M, Wiche G. Conditional targeting of plectin in prenatal and adult mouse stratified epithelia causes keratinocyte fragility and lesional epidermal barrier defects. J Cell Sci. 2007;120(Pt 14):2435-2443.

[23] Guo L, Degenstein L, Dowling J, Yu QC, Wollmann R, Perman B, Fuchs E. Gene targeting of BPAG1: abnormalities in mechanical strength and cell migration in stratified epithelia and neurologic degeneration. Cell. 1995;81(2):233-243.

[24] Gallicano GI, Kouklis P, Bauer C, Yin M, Vasioukhin V, Degenstein L, Fuchs E. Desmoplakin is required early in development for assembly of desmosomes and cytoskeletal linkage. J Cell Biol. 1998;143(7):2009-2022.

[25] Vasioukhin V, Bowers E, Bauer C, Degenstein L, Fuchs E. Desmoplakin is essential in epidermal sheet formation. Nat Cell Biol. 2001;3(12):1076-1085.

[26] Bierkamp C, McLaughlin KJ, Schwarz H, Huber O, Kemler R. Embryonic heart and skin defects in mice lacking plakoglobin. Dev Biol. 1996;180(2):780-785.

[27] Dowling J, Yu QC, Fuchs E. Beta4 integrin is required for hemidesmosome formation, cell adhesion and cell survival. J Cell Biol. 1996;134(2):559-572.

[28] van der Neut R, Krimpenfort P, Calafat J, Niessen CM, Sonnenberg A. Epithelial detachment due to absence of hemidesmosomes in integrin beta 4 null mice. Nat Genet. 1996;13(3):366-369.

[29] Murgia C, Blaikie P, Kim N, Dans M, Petrie HT, Giancotti FG. Cell cycle and adhesion defects in mice carrying a targeted deletion of the integrin beta4 cytoplasmic domain. Embo J. 1998;17(14):3940-3951.

[30] Raymond K, Kreft M, Janssen H, Calafat J, Sonnenberg A. Keratinocytes display normal proliferation, survival and differentiation in conditional beta4-integrin knockout mice. J Cell Sci. 2005;118(Pt 5):1045-1060.

[31] Nishie W, Sawamura D, Goto M, Ito K, Shibaki A, McMillan JR, Sakai K, Nakamura H, Olasz E, Yancey KB, Akiyama M, Shimizu H. Humanization of autoantigen. Nat Med. 2007;13(3):378-383.

[32] Coulombe PA, Lee CH. Defining keratin protein function in skin epithelia: epidermolysis bullosa simplex and its aftermath. J Invest Dermatol. 2012;132(3 Pt 2):763-775.

[33] Schweizer J, Bowden PE, Coulombe PA, Langbein L, Lane EB, Magin TM, Maltais L, Omary MB, Parry DAD, Rogers MA, Wright MW. New consensus nomenclature for mammalian keratins. J Cell Biol. 2006;174(2):169-174.

[34] Moll R, Franke WW, Schiller DL, Geiger B, Krepler R. The catalog of human cytokeratins: patterns of expression in normal epithelia, tumors and cultured cells. Cell. 1982;31(1):11-24.

[35] Nelson WG, Sun TT. The 50- and 58-kdalton keratin classes as molecular markers for stratified squamous epithelia: cell culture studies. J Cell Biol. 1983;97(1):244-251.

[36] Kitajima Y, Inoue S, Yaoita H. Abnormal organization of keratin intermediate filaments in cultured keratinocytes of epidermolysis bullosa simplex. Arch Dermatol Res. 1989;281(1):5-10.

[37] Anton-Lamprecht I, Schnyder UW. Epidermolysis bullosa herpetiformis Dowling-Meara. Report of a case and pathomorphogenesis. Dermatologica. 1982;164(4):221-235.

[38] Bonifas JM, Rothman AL, Epstein EH, Jr. Epidermolysis bullosa simplex: evidence in two families for keratin gene abnormalities. Science. 1991;254(5035):1202-1205.

[39] Coulombe PA, Hutton ME, Letai A, Hebert A, Paller AS, Fuchs E. Point mutations in human keratin 14 genes of epidermolysis bullosa simplex patients: genetic and functional analyses. Cell. 1991;66(6):1301-1311.

[40] Lane EB, Rugg EL, Navsaria H, Leigh IM, Heagerty AH, Ishida-Yamamoto A, Eady RA. A mutation in the conserved helix termination peptide of keratin 5 in hereditary skin blistering. Nature. 1992;356(6366):244-246.

[41] Szeverenyi I, Cassidy AJ, Chung CW, Lee BT, Common JE, Ogg SC, Chen H, Sim SY, Goh WL, Ng KW, Simpson JA, Chee LL, Eng GH, Li B, Lunny DP, Chuon D, Venkatesh A, Khoo KH, McLean WH, Lim YP, Lane EB. The Human Intermediate Filament Database: comprehensive information on a gene family involved in many human diseases. Hum Mutat. 2008;29(3):351-360.

[42] Ishida-Yamamoto A, McGrath JA, Chapman SJ, Leigh IM, Lane EB, Eady RA. Epidermolysis bullosa simplex (Dowling-Meara type) is a genetic disease characterized by an abnormal keratin-filament network involving keratins K5 and K14. J Invest Dermatol. 1991;97(6):959-968.

[43] Cummins RE, Klingberg S, Wesley J, Rogers M, Zhao Y, Murrell DF. Keratin 14 point mutations at codon 119 of helix 1A resulting in different epidermolysis bullosa simplex phenotypes. J Invest Dermatol. 2001;117(5):1103-1107.

[44] Natsuga K, Nishie W, Smith BJ, Shinkuma S, Smith TA, Parry DA, Oiso N, Kawada A, Yoneda K, Akiyama M, Shimizu H. Consequences of two different amino-acid substitutions at the same codon in KRT14 indicate definitive roles of structural distortion in epidermolysis bullosa simplex pathogenesis. J Invest Dermatol. 2011;131(9):1869-1876.

[45] Sorensen CB, Andresen BS, Jensen UB, Jensen TG, Jensen PK, Gregersen N, Bolund L. Functional testing of keratin 14 mutant proteins associated with the three major subtypes of epidermolysis bullosa simplex. Exp Dermatol. 2003;12(4):472-479.

[46] Atkinson SD, McGilligan VE, Liao H, Szeverenyi I, Smith FJ, Moore CB, McLean WH. Development of allele-specific therapeutic siRNA for keratin 5 mutations in epidermolysis bullosa simplex. J Invest Dermatol. 2011;131(10):2079-2086.

[47] Natsuga K, Nishie W, Akiyama M, Nakamura H, Shinkuma S, McMillan JR, Nagasaki A, Has C, Ouchi T, Ishiko A, Hirako Y, Owaribe K, Sawamura D, Bruckner-Tuderman L, Shimizu H. Plectin expression patterns determine two distinct subtypes of epidermolysis bullosa simplex. Hum Mutat. 2010;31(3):308-316.

[48] Natsuga K, Nishie W, Shinkuma S, Arita K, Nakamura H, Ohyama M, Osaka H, Kambara T, Hirako Y, Shimizu H. Plectin deficiency leads to both muscular dystrophy and pyloric atresia in epidermolysis bullosa simplex. Hum Mutat. 2010;31(10):E1687-1698.

[49] Kiritsi D, Pigors M, Tantcheva-Poor I, Wessel C, Arin MJ, Kohlhase J, Bruckner-Tuderman L, Has C. Epidermolysis Bullosa Simplex Ogna Revisited. J Invest Dermatol. 2012.

[50] Fuchs P, Zorer M, Rezniczek GA, Spazierer D, Oehler S, Castanon MJ, Hauptmann R, Wiche G. Unusual 5' transcript complexity of plectin isoforms: novel tissue-specific exons modulate actin binding activity. Hum Mol Genet. 1999;8(13):2461-2472.

[51] Andra K, Kornacker I, Jorgl A, Zorer M, Spazierer D, Fuchs P, Fischer I, Wiche G. Plectin-isoform-specific rescue of hemidesmosomal defects in plectin (-/-) keratinocytes. J Invest Dermatol. 2003;120(2):189-197.

[52] Elliott CE, Becker B, Oehler S, Castanon MJ, Hauptmann R, Wiche G. Plectin transcript diversity: identification and tissue distribution of variants with distinct first coding exons and rodless isoforms. Genomics. 1997;42(1):115-125.

[53] McLean WH, Pulkkinen L, Smith FJ, Rugg EL, Lane EB, Bullrich F, Burgeson RE, Amano S, Hudson DL, Owaribe K, McGrath JA, McMillan JR, Eady RA, Leigh IM, Christiano AM, Uitto J. Loss of plectin causes epidermolysis bullosa with muscular dystrophy: cDNA cloning and genomic organization. Genes Dev. 1996;10(14):1724-1735.

[54] Smith FJ, Eady RA, Leigh IM, McMillan JR, Rugg EL, Kelsell DP, Bryant SP, Spurr NK, Geddes JF, Kirtschig G, Milana G, de Bono AG, Owaribe K, Wiche G, Pulkkinen L, Uitto J, McLean WH, Lane EB. Plectin deficiency results in muscular dystrophy with epidermolysis bullosa. Nat Genet. 1996;13(4):450-457.

[55] Sonnenberg A, Liem RK. Plakins in development and disease. Exp Cell Res. 2007;313(10):2189-2203.

[56] Nakamura H, Sawamura D, Goto M, Nakamura H, McMillan JR, Park S, Kono S, Hasegawa S, Paku S, Nakamura T, Ogiso Y, Shimizu H. Epidermolysis bullosa simplex associated with pyloric atresia is a novel clinical subtype caused by mutations in the plectin gene (PLEC1). J Mol Diagn. 2005;7(1):28-35.

[57] Pfendner E, Uitto J. Plectin gene mutations can cause epidermolysis bullosa with pyloric atresia. J Invest Dermatol. 2005;124(1):111-115.

[58] Vidal F, Aberdam D, Miquel C, Christiano AM, Pulkkinen L, Uitto J, Ortonne JP, Meneguzzi G. Integrin beta 4 mutations associated with junctional epidermolysis bullosa with pyloric atresia. Nat Genet. 1995;10(2):229-234.

[59] Ruzzi L, Gagnoux-Palacios L, Pinola M, Belli S, Meneguzzi G, D'Alessio M, Zambruno G. A homozygous mutation in the integrin alpha6 gene in junctional epidermolysis bullosa with pyloric atresia. J Clin Invest. 1997;99(12):2826-2831.

[60] Koss-Harnes D, Hoyheim B, Anton-Lamprecht I, Gjesti A, Jorgensen RS, Jahnsen FL, Olaisen B, Wiche G, Gedde-Dahl T, Jr. A site-specific plectin mutation causes dominant epidermolysis bullosa simplex Ogna: two identical de novo mutations. J Invest Dermatol. 2002;118(1):87-93.

[61] Labib RS, Anhalt GJ, Patel HP, Mutasim DF, Diaz LA. Molecular heterogeneity of the bullous pemphigoid antigens as detected by immunoblotting. J Immunol. 1986;136(4):1231-1235.

[62] Sawamura D, Li K, Chu ML, Uitto J. Human bullous pemphigoid antigen (BPAG1). Amino acid sequences deduced from cloned cDNAs predict biologically important peptide segments and protein domains. J Biol Chem. 1991;266(27):17784-17790.

[63] Giudice GJ, Emery DJ, Diaz LA. Cloning and primary structural analysis of the bullous pemphigoid autoantigen BP180. J Invest Dermatol. 1992;99(3):243-250.

[64] McGrath JA, Gatalica B, Christiano AM, Li K, Owaribe K, McMillan JR, Eady RA, Uitto J. Mutations in the 180-kD bullous pemphigoid antigen (BPAG2), a hemidesmosomal transmembrane collagen (COL17A1), in generalized atrophic benign epidermolysis bullosa. Nat Genet. 1995;11(1):83-86.

[65] Green KJ, Goldman RD, Chisholm RL. Isolation of cDNAs encoding desmosomal plaque proteins: evidence that bovine desmoplakins I and II are derived from two mRNAs and a single gene. Proc Natl Acad Sci U S A. 1988;85(8):2613-2617.

[66] Uzumcu A, Norgett EE, Dindar A, Uyguner O, Nisli K, Kayserili H, Sahin SE, Dupont E, Severs NJ, Leigh IM, Yuksel-Apak M, Kelsell DP, Wollnik B. Loss of desmoplakin isoform I causes early onset cardiomyopathy and heart failure in a Naxos-like syndrome. J Med Genet. 2006;43(2):e5.

[67] Anhalt GJ, Kim SC, Stanley JR, Korman NJ, Jabs DA, Kory M, Izumi H, Ratrie H, 3rd, Mutasim D, Ariss-Abdo L, et al. Paraneoplastic pemphigus. An autoimmune mucocutaneous disease associated with neoplasia. N Engl J Med. 1990;323(25):1729-1735.

[68] Oursler JR, Labib RS, Ariss-Abdo L, Burke T, O'Keefe EJ, Anhalt GJ. Human autoantibodies against desmoplakins in paraneoplastic pemphigus. J Clin Invest. 1992;89(6):1775-1782.

[69] Bolling MC, Jonkman MF. Skin and heart: une liaison dangereuse. Exp Dermatol. 2009;18(8):658-668.

[70] Jonkman MF, Pasmooij AM, Pasmans SG, van den Berg MP, Ter Horst HJ, Timmer A, Pas HH. Loss of desmoplakin tail causes lethal acantholytic epidermolysis bullosa. Am J Hum Genet. 2005;77(4):653-660.

[71] Bolling MC, Veenstra MJ, Jonkman MF, Diercks GF, Curry CJ, Fisher J, Pas HH, Bruckner AL. Lethal acantholytic epidermolysis bullosa due to a novel homozygous deletion in DSP: expanding the phenotype and implications for desmoplakin function in skin and heart. Br J Dermatol. 2010;162(6):1388-1394.

[72] Hobbs RP, Han SY, van der Zwaag PA, Bolling MC, Jongbloed JD, Jonkman MF, Getsios S, Paller AS, Green KJ. Insights from a desmoplakin mutation identified in lethal acantholytic epidermolysis bullosa. J Invest Dermatol. 2010;130(11):2680-2683.

[73] McGrath JA, McMillan JR, Shemanko CS, Runswick SK, Leigh IM, Lane EB, Garrod DR, Eady RA. Mutations in the plakophilin 1 gene result in ectodermal dysplasia/skin fragility syndrome. Nat Genet. 1997;17(2):240-244.

[74] Wolf A, Krause-Gruszczynska M, Birkenmeier O, Ostareck-Lederer A, Huttelmaier S, Hatzfeld M. Plakophilin 1 stimulates translation by promoting eIF4A1 activity. J Cell Biol. 2010;188(4):463-471.

Chapter 3

Junctional and Dystrophic Epidermolysis Bullosa

Daisuke Tsuruta, Chiharu Tateishi and Masamitsu Ishii

Additional information is available at the end of the chapter

http://dx.doi.org/10.5772/54610

1. Introduction

Epidermolysis bullosa (EB) is a congenital genodermatosis, which affects mainly skin and occasionally other organs [1]. Lifelong blistering and erosion of the skin and mucous membrane, caused by mechanical trauma, threaten EB patients [1]. The most common cause of death is metastasizing squamous cell carcinoma [2]. EB is subdivided into mainly three categories by the location of tissue separation (blister) in the basement membrane zone (BMZ) at the electronmicroscopical level, EB simplex (EBS), dystrophic EB (DEB) and junctional EB (JEB)[1]. Some dermatologists also proposed to distinguish hemidesmosomal epidermolysis bullosa [3]. In EBS, blister locates at the level of basal keratinocytes, in DEB at the level of lamina lucida and in DEB at the level of the dermis [1]. EB is mainly caused by the mutation of keratin filament, hemidesmosome components or collagen genes [1]. Thus far, at least 10 different genes are identified as causative genes for EB [1,4,5].

2. The molecular components of BMZ (Figure 1)

The keratin is the most abundant structural proteins found in epithelial cells [6]. The keratins are polymers of type I and type II intermediate filaments [6]. In basal keratinocytes, type I intermediate filament is keratin 14 (K14) and type II intermediate filament is keratin 5 (K5)[6]. These two types of keratins are the major mutated molecules found in EBS [6].

Hemidesmosomes are very tight cell-matrix junction structures which connect basal keratinocytes to the basement membrane [7]. Hemidesmosomes tether keratin filaments to the cell surface [7]. Ultrastructurally, hemidemosomes comprises the inner plaques, the outer plaques, anchoring fibrils and anchoring filaments [8]. At the molecular level, core of each hemidesmosome comprises of four transmembrane proteins, 180 kDa-bullous pemphigoid antigen (BP180, type XVII collagen, BPAG2), α6β4 integrins and CD151 tetraspanin protein [7]. Both BP180 and α6β4 integrin interacts with laminin-332 at the BMZ

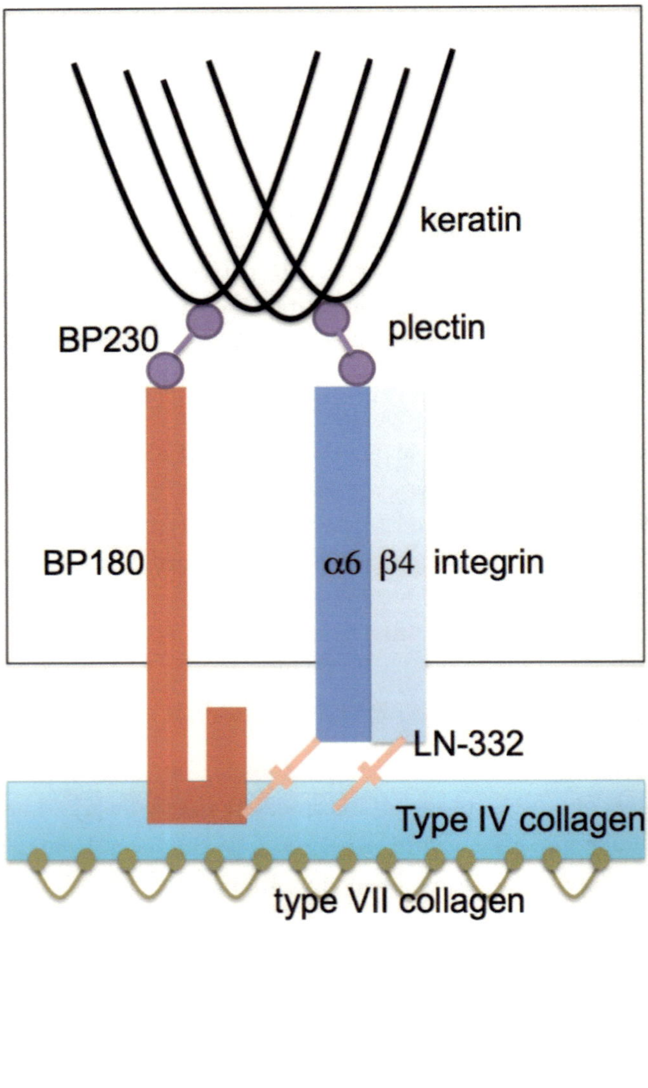

Figure 1. Molecular components of basement membrane zone.

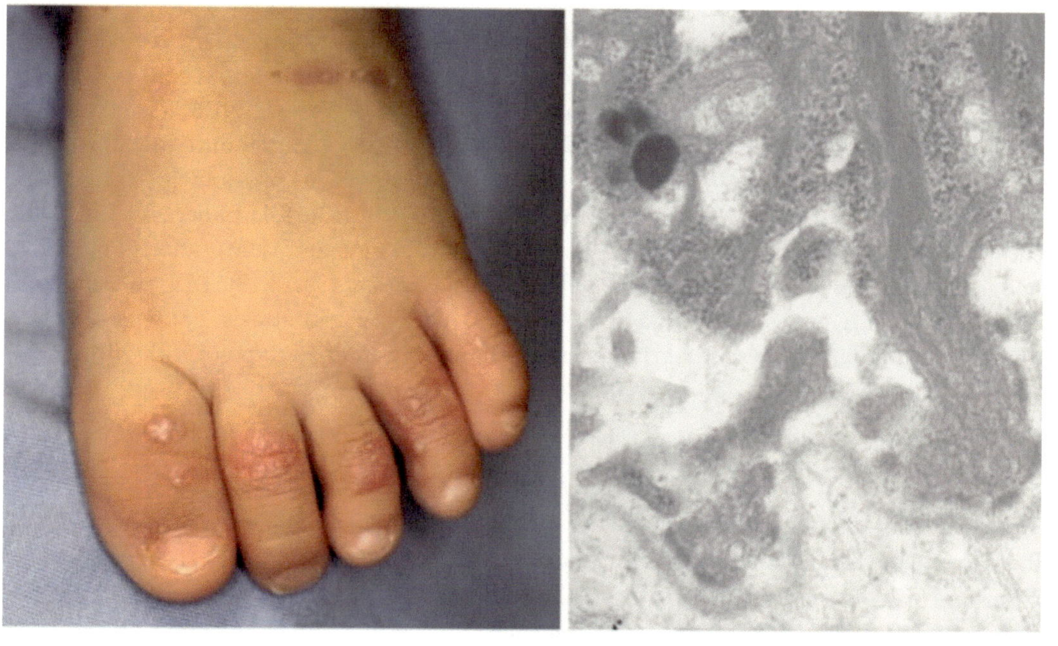

Figure 2. Clinical (left) and electronmicroscopical (right) appearances of dystrophic epidermolysis bullosa patient.

[9]. $\alpha 6\beta 4$ integrin is the unique integrin, because the other integrins normally attach to actin, while $\alpha 6\beta 4$ integrin attaches to intermediate filament, keratin [10]. $\alpha 6\beta 4$ integrin attaches to intermediate filament by plectin [10]. BP180 tethers keratin through the interaction with BP230 in the cytoplasm [10]. Both BP180 and BP230 are the target of major subepidermal autoimmune bullous disease, bullous pemphigoid [11]. Basement membrane is mainly composed of collagen IV [12]. Laminin-332 and collagen VII adhere to collagen IV [7]. All these components are molecules which are affected by EB patients [1].

3. JEB (Figure 2)

The manner of inheritance in JEB patients is autosomal recessive [1]. As mentioned above, skin separation in JEB occurs in the lamina lucida [1]. Three subtypes of JEB exsist, Herlitz JEB, non-Herlitz JEB and JEB with pyloric atresia [1]. Herlitz JEB is fatal subtype of JEB [1]. Most affected patients die from systemic infection through severe erosion on virtually entire skin [1]. Herlitz JEB is caused by homozygous or compound heterozygous premature termination codon (PTC) mutation of laminin-332 [13,14]. Non-Herlitz JEB is much milder than Herlitz JEB [1]. Either missense mutation of laminin-332 or mutation of BP180 is found in non-Herlitz JEB patients [15-17]. JEB with pyloric atresia is possibly life-threatening subtype, similar to Herlitz JEB [1]. However, JEB with pyloric atresia patients occasionally show non-life-threatening phenotype like non-Herlitz JEB patients [1]. Mutations in $\alpha 6$ or $\beta 4$ integrin genes are found in JEB with pyloric atresia patients [1,18,19]. PTC mutations of $\alpha 6$ or $\beta 4$ integrin genes are found in severe JEB with pyloric atresia patients, whereas missense mutations of these integrin genes are found in milder subtype of JEB with pyloric atresia patients [1,20].

4. DEB

Tissue separation of DEB occurs in the dermis [1]. Clinically, DEB patients show blistering of the skin in the large area along with scarring and milia formation [15]. Two fashions of inheritance are known in DEB, autosomal dominant and autosomal recessive [15]. DEB is known to be caused by mutations in collagen VII gene. More than 300 mutations are reported in DEB [15]. Glycine substitution mutation in one allele of gene encoding the collagenous domain of collagen VII is known to be strongly associated with DEB [21]. Such mutation probably has a dominant negative effect on collagen VII formation or assembly [15]. In the severest form of DEB, Hallopeau-Siemens recessive DEB, PTC mutation on both alleles of gene encoding collagen VII is found [22]. In the mildest form of recessive DEB, non-Hallopeau-Siemens recessive DEB, PTC mutations in one allele, missense or in-frame mutations are found in the genes encoding collagen VII [23].

5. Diagnosis

The hallmark of the diagnosis of EB is made by DNA-based mutational analysis [1]. However, it is required to minimize the effort to specify the possible affected gene through history taking, clinical assessment, histopathological study, immunomapping study and electronmicroscopic study [1]. Using these methods, we can categorize the disease type of patients into at least three forms, EBS, JEB and DEB [1]. Histopathology or electronmicroscopy samples should be taken after gentle rubbing on non-blistered skin, in order not to misdiagnose the location of blister by degeneration of the affected skin [1]. Immunomapping study using anti-K5, K14, α6 integrin, β4 integrin, BP180, plectin, laminin-332 or collagen VII antibody is quite useful to diagnose EB, if the affected mutation locates on the portion of epitope targeted by these antibodies [1]. In addition, immunohistochemical study using anti-collagen IV antibody is also useful to assess the portion of the split [1]. In EBS or JEB sample, positive staining of collagen IV is found at the floor of the blister, whereas in DEB sample, that is found at the roof of the blister [1]. After these careful assessments, DNA-based diagnoses are performed [1].

6. Treatment

Treatment of EB is mainly symptomatic one. Most important issue is to prevent local infection, including Staphylococcus aureus, Streptococcus pyogenes and Psudomonas aeruginosa. If we fail to control local infection, subsequent sepsis occurs with high possibility. In order to prevent such local infection, semiocclusive nonadherent dressings with or without topical antibiotics is selected for the treatment of EB. In addition, as esophageal ocular and oral complications are also found in EB patients, clinical care for erosions in these organs are also required to prevent local infection and resultant sepsis.

Allogeneic skin grafts, in which cells do not derived from patients, were tried for EB patients. These allografts were rejected but could produce cytokines to facilitate the wound healing and re-epithelization process.

7. Ongoing therapies

As symptomatic therapy is only available for EB, future gene-targeted therapy is highly expected and is being considered. To attempt to do so, cell-based therapies using fibroblasts and allogeneic bone marrow transplantation are the potential options. As the experimental level, such therapies were successful for JEB and DEB. Collgen VII is known to be synthesized mainly by keratinocytes and to a lesser extent by fibroblasts [19]. As fibroblasts are easy to culture and easy to get transfected by external genes than keratinocytes, cell-based therapies using fibroblasts are selected for the possible gene therapy for DEB [1]. In fact, Goto et al. successfully restores collagen VII by skin collagen VII gene transfected fibroblast introduction [24]. In addition, clinical study for five patients using this technique was already successful without any adverse effects [25]. Cultured patient keratinocytes transfected with laminin β3 gene through retroviral technique were successfully transferred and healed blister formation in one patient. Collagen VII protein therapy was also introduced and was successful in an in vivo model. The missing or defective protein, synthesized by in vitro recombinant methods, is introduced to blistered skin. Successful treatment was already obtained in case of collagen VII [26,27].

Allogeneic bone marrow transplantation is the other option. In EB patients, basal keratinocytes produce defective gene product of BMZ [1]. It is known that, bone marrow cells have a potential to differentiate into epidermal keratinocytes [17]. Therefore, allogeneic bone marrow transplantation can correct such defective BMZ components. As an experimental level, Chino et al. was successful in correcting ameliorated collagen VII in collagen VII knock out mice by allogeneic bone marrow transplantation [28]. Moreover, clinical trial using this technology and cord blood transplantation were already started and were obtained successful results [1].

8. Conclusion

EB is a life-threatening and life-long disease with only symptomatic treatments, thus far. However, cell-based gene-targeting therapy is on the way to be successful.

Author details

Daisuke Tsuruta*, Chiharu Tateishi and Masamitsu Ishii
Department of Dermatology, Osaka City University Graduate School of Medicine, Osaka, Japan

9. References

[1] Sawamura D, Nakano H, Matsuzaki Y. Overview of epidermolysis bullosa. J Dermatol. 2010;37:214-219.
[2] Salas-Alanis JC, Cepeda-Valdes R, Mellerio JE, Christiano AM, Uitto J. Progress in epidermolysis bullosa: summary of a workshop in CILAD-2010*. Int J Dermatol. 2012;51:682-687.
[3] Pai S, Marinkovich MP. Epidermolysis bullosa: new and emerging trends. Am J Clin Dermatol. 2002;3:371-380.
[4] Pulkkinen L, Marinkovich MP, Tran HT, Lin L, Herron GS, Uitto J. Compound heterozygosity for novel splice site mutations in the BPAG2/COL17A1 gene underlies generalized atrophic benign epidermolysis bullosa. J Invest Dermatol. 1999;113:1114-1118.
[5] Uitto J, Richard G. Progress in epidermolysis bullosa: from eponyms to molecular genetic classification. Clin Dermatol. 2005;23:33-40.
[6] Coulombe PA, Lee CH. Defining keratin protein function in skin epithelia: epidermolysis bullosa simplex and its aftermath. J Invest Dermatol. 2012;132(3 Pt 2):763-775.

---

* Corresponding Author

[7] Tsuruta D, Hashimoto T, Hamill KJ, Jones JC. Hemidesmosomes and focal contact proteins: functions and cross-talk in keratinocytes, bullous diseases and wound healing. J Dermatol Sci. 2011;62:1-7.

[8] Shinkuma S, McMillan JR, Shimizu H. Ultrastructure and molecular pathogenesis of epidermolysis bullosa. Clin Dermatol. 2011;29:412-419.

[9] Tsuruta D, Kobayashi H, Imanishi H, Sugawara K, Ishii M, Jones JC. Laminin-332-integrin interaction: a target for cancer therapy? Curr Med Chem. 2008;15:1968-1975.

[10] Jones JC, Hopkinson SB, Goldfinger LE. Structure and assembly of hemidesmosomes. BioEssays. 1998;20:488-494.

[11] Ujiie H, Shibaki A, Nishie W, Shimizu H. What's new in bullous pemphigoid. J Dermatol. 2010;37:194-204.

[12] Abreu-Velez AM, Howard MS. Collagen IV in Normal Skin and in Pathological Processes. North Am J Med Sci. 2012;4:1-8.

[13] Pulkkinen L, Christiano AM, Airenne T, Haakana H, Tryggvason K, Uitto J. Mutations in the gamma 2 chain gene (LAMC2) of kalinin/laminin 5 in the junctional forms of epidermolysis bullosa. Nat Genet. 1994;6:293-297.

[14] Aberdam D, Galliano MF, Vailly J, Pulkkinen L, Bonifas J, Christiano AM, et al. Herlitz's junctional epidermolysis bullosa is linked to mutations in the gene (LAMC2) for the gamma 2 subunit of nicein/kalinin (LAMININ-5). Nat Genet. 1994;6:299-304.

[15] McGrath JA, Pulkkinen L, Christiano AM, Leigh IM, Eady RA, Uitto J. Altered laminin 5 expression due to mutations in the gene encoding the beta 3 chain (LAMB3) in generalized atrophic benign epidermolysis bullosa. J Invest Dermatol. 1995;104:467-474.

[16] McGrath JA, Gatalica B, Christiano AM, Li K, Owaribe K, McMillan JR, et al. Mutations in the 180-kD bullous pemphigoid antigen (BPAG2), a hemidesmosomal transmembrane collagen (COL17A1), in generalized atrophic benign epidermolysis bullosa. Nat Genet. 1995;11:83-86.

[17] Nishie W, Sawamura D, Goto M, Ito K, Shibaki A, McMillan JR, et al. Humanization of autoantigen. Nat Med. 2007;13:378-383.

[18] Vidal F, Aberdam D, Miquel C, Christiano AM, Pulkkinen L, Uitto J, et al. Integrin beta 4 mutations associated with junctional epidermolysis bullosa with pyloric atresia. Nat Genet. 1995;10:229-234.

[19] Georges-Labouesse E, Messaddeq N, Yehia G, Cadalbert L, Dierich A, Le Meur M. Absence of integrin alpha 6 leads to epidermolysis bullosa and neonatal death in mice. Nat Genet. 1996;13:370-373.

[20] Abe M, Sawamura D, Goto M, Nakamura H, Nagasaki A, Nomura Y, et al. ITGB4 missense mutation in a transmembrane domain causes non-lethal variant of junctional epidermolysis bullosa with pyloric atresia. J Dermatol Sci. 2007;47:165-167.

[21] Christiano AM, Ryynanen M, Uitto J. Dominant dystrophic epidermolysis bullosa: identification of a Gly-->Ser substitution in the triple-helical domain of type VII collagen. Proc Nat Acad Sci. 1994;91:3549-3553.

[22] Hilal L, Rochat A, Duquesnoy P, Blanchet-Bardon C, Wechsler J, Martin N, et al. A homozygous insertion-deletion in the type VII collagen gene (COL7A1) in Hallopeau-Siemens dystrophic epidermolysis bullosa. Natu Genet. 1993;5:287-293.

[23] Christiano AM, Greenspan DS, Hoffman GG, Zhang X, Tamai Y, Lin AN, et al. A missense mutation in type VII collagen in two affected siblings with recessive dystrophic epidermolysis bullosa. Nat Genet. 1993;4:62-66.

[24] Goto M, Sawamura D, Ito K, Abe M, Nishie W, Sakai K, et al. Fibroblasts show more potential as target cells than keratinocytes in COL7A1 gene therapy of dystrophic epidermolysis bullosa. J Invest Dermatol. 2006;126:766-772.

[25] Wong T, Gammon L, Liu L, Mellerio JE, Dopping-Hepenstal PJ, Pacy J, et al. Potential of fibroblast cell therapy for recessive dystrophic epidermolysis bullosa. J Invest Dermatol. 2008;128:2179-2189.

[26] Woodley DT, Keene DR, Atha T, Huang Y, Ram R, Kasahara N, et al.Intradermal injection of lentiviral vectors corrects regenerated human dystrophic epidermolysis bullosa skin tissue in vivo. Molecular therapy : J Am Soc Gen Ther. 2004;10:318-326.

[27] Woodley DT, Keene DR, Atha T, Huang Y, Lipman K, Li W, et al. Injection of recombinant human type VII collagen restores collagen function in dystrophic epidermolysis bullosa. Nat Med. 2004;10:693-695.

[28] Chino T, Tamai K, Yamazaki T, Otsuru S, Kikuchi Y, Nimura K, et al. Bonemarrow cell transfer into fetal circulation can ameliorate genetic skin diseases by providing fibroblasts to the skin and inducing immune tolerance. Am J Pathol. 2008;173:803-814.

Chapter 4

Hereditary Palmoplantar Keratosis

Tamihiro Kawakami

Additional information is available at the end of the chapter

http://dx.doi.org/10.5772/53572

1. Introduction

Palmoplantar keratosis or palmoplantar keratoderma (PPK) constitutes a heterogeneous group of disorders characterized by excessive epidermal thickening of the palms and soles of affected individuals [1]. PPK can be characterized as either inherited or acquired. Transgredient PPK extends beyond palmoplantar skin, contiguously or as callosities on pressure points on the fingers or knuckles, or elsewhere. Typical pathohistological findings of PPK are orthokeratotic hyperkeratosis, hyper- or hypogranulosis and acanthosis. These changes are non-specific and found in many types of PPK.

PPK is classified clinically as diffuse, focal, striate, or punctuate and develops either in isolation or in association with other cutaneous or extracutaneous manifestations. The diffuse type consists of uniform involvement of the palmoplantar surface. The focal type consists of localized areas of hyperkeratosis located mainly on pressure points and sites of recurrent friction. The striate type presents with linear hyperkeratosis on the palms and soles. The punctate type features multiple small, hyperkeratotic papules, spicules, or nodules on the palms and soles. These tiny keratoses may involve the entire palmoplantar surface or may be restricted to certain locations.

2. Diffuse PPK

2.1. Unna-Thost PPK

Unna-Thost PPK is inherited in an autosomally dominant manner without associated organ involvement. The condition may manifest in the first few months of life but is usually well developed by age 3-4 years. The disease develops in early childhood and persists throughout life. Clinically, there is hyperkeratosis on the palms and soles. Unna-Thost PPK is characterized by a well-demarcated, symmetric, often "waxy" hyperkeratosis involving the whole of the palms and soles. It is usually nontransgredient, with a sharp demarcation of the lesions at the wrists. Aberrant keratotic lesions may appear in the dorsum of the hands, feet, knees, and elbows. The dorsa of the fingers may be involved with a sclerodermalike thickening of the distal digit. A cobblestone hyperkeratosis of the knuckles may be seen. Nails may be thickened.

Histological findings include orthokeratotic hyperkeratosis associated with hypergranulosis or hypogranulosis and moderate acanthosis. Molecular biology features include linkage to type II keratin locus on band 12q11-13, corresponding to a keratin 1 gene mutation. Treatment includes salicylic acid, 50% propylene glycol in water under plastic occlusion several nights per week, and lactic acid- and urea-containing creams and lotions; all have been shown to be helpful. Mechanical debridement with a blade may also be useful. Oral retinoid therapy has had variable effects.

2.2. Vörner PPK

This type is inherited in an autosomal dominant fashion. It has an estimated prevalence of at least 4.4 cases per 100,000 population in Northern Ireland. Onset occurs in the first few months of life, but the disease is usually well developed by age 3-4 years. A well-demarcated, symmetric thick, yellow hyperkeratosis is present over the palms and soles, often with a "dirty" snakeskin appearance due to underlying epidermolysis [2]. An erythematous band is frequently present at the periphery of the keratosis. The surface is often uneven and verrucous. Finally, it is usually nontransgredient, with a sharp demarcation of the lesions at the wrists.

Histologically, keratinocytes show epidermolysis, hyperkeratosis, acanthosis, and papillomatosis. Perinuclear vacuolization and large keratohyalin granules are seen. Cellular breakdown in the spinous and granular cell layers sometimes leads to blister formation. Keratin 1 and keratin 9 mutations have also been reported. Treatment includes salicylic acid, 50% propylene glycol in water under plastic occlusion several nights per week, and lactic acid- and urea-containing creams and lotions; all have been shown to be helpful. Mechanical debridement with a blade also may be useful. Oral retinoid therapy has had variable effects and may not benefit patients with certain genotype profiles, such as K1 mutations.

Clinical features of Vörner PPK are very similiar to Unna-Thost PPK. Unna-Thost PPK may have a waxy appearance, compared with the dirty appearance of Vörner PPK. Hyperhidrosis and pitted keratolysis may be present with Unna-Thost PPK. Differentiation from Unna-Thost PPK can be made histopathologically, with the finding of epidermolysis. There is no epidermolysis or vacuolar changes in Unna-Thost PPK.

2.3. Mal de Meleda

Mal de Meleda is characterized by a diffuse, thick hyperkeratosis with a prominent erythematous border. This disease is characterized by early infancy onset and follows a progressive course with extension to the dorsal surfaces of the hands and feet. This condition is inherited in an autosomal recessive fashion. The prevalence is 1 case per 100,000 population. The disease has its onset in early infancy and follows a progressive course. It was first described in inhabitants of the Adriatic Island of Meleda.

Mal de Meleda frequently presents with constrictive bands, perioral erythema, nail changes, and occasional brachydactyly, with a progressive clinical course throughout the patients' lives. The main clinical characteristics are transgressive PPK, hyperhidrosis, and perioral erythema. Clinical dermatological features include diffuse, thick keratoderma with a prominent erythematous border. Lesions spread onto the dorsa of the hands and the feet (transgredient). Constricting bands are present around the digits and can result in spontaneous amputation. Well-circumscribed psoriasis-like plaques or lichenoid patches may be present on the knees and the elbows. Patients may have severe hyperhidrosis, possibly accompanied by malodor. Secondary bacterial and fungal infections are common. Other clinical features include: lingua plicata, syndactyly, hair on the palms and the soles, high-arched palate, and left-handedness.

Histologic findings include orthokeratosis and normogranulosis without epidermolysis. Mutations in the gene SLURP1 located on chromosome 8q24.3 were identified as the cause of Mal de Meleda. Molecular biology features include mutations in the gene encoding SLURP1 found on band 8q24.3.

2.4. Nagashima-type PPK

Nagashima-type PPK is included in the diffuse autosomal recessive type of hereditary PPKs without associated features [3]. Nagashima-type PPK was first described in a report from Japan in 1977. Since then, more than 20 cases have been reported in Japan. Nagashima-type cases have been reported only in the Japanese literature; this type of PPK is not well known in Western countries, even though the existence of this disease is recognized. Therefore, the definition and characterization of this disease have not been well recognized globally.

Onset of disease occurs between birth and age 3 years (Figures 1, 2). Because its clinical manifestations are similar to but milder than those of mal de Meleda, it was originally described as a mild form of Mal de Meleda. Mal de Meleda is much more severe than Nagashima-type. It usually involves perioral erythema and occasionally exhibits brachydactyly, nail abnormalities, and lichenoid plaques. Unlike Mal de Meleda, spontaneous amputation has never been observed in Nagashima type PPK. Furthermore, there is no evidence of a SLURP1 mutation in patients with Nagashima-type PPK. The results of genetic study suggested that Nagashima-type PPK is distinct from Mal de Meleda.

2.5. Vohwinkel syndrome

Vohwinkel syndrome (mutilating and diffuse PPK) is associated with various extracutaneous features, including ichthyosis and deafness. Onset occurs in infancy. Clinically, this condition manifests in infants as a honeycomblike keratosis of the palms and the soles. It becomes transgredient during childhood. Later-forming, constricting, fibrous bands appear on the digits and can lead to progressive strangulation and autoamputation. Starfish-shaped keratosis may occur on the knuckles of the fingers and toes, which is a characteristic feature of this disorder. Alopecia, hearing loss, spastic paraplegia, myopathy, ichthyosiform dermatosis, and nail abnormalities are other associated manifestations. Other reported findings are deaf-mutism, congenital alopecia universalis, pseudopelade type alopecia, acanthosis nigricans, spastic paraplegia, myopathy, nail changes, mental retardation, bullous lesions on the soles, and seizures [4].

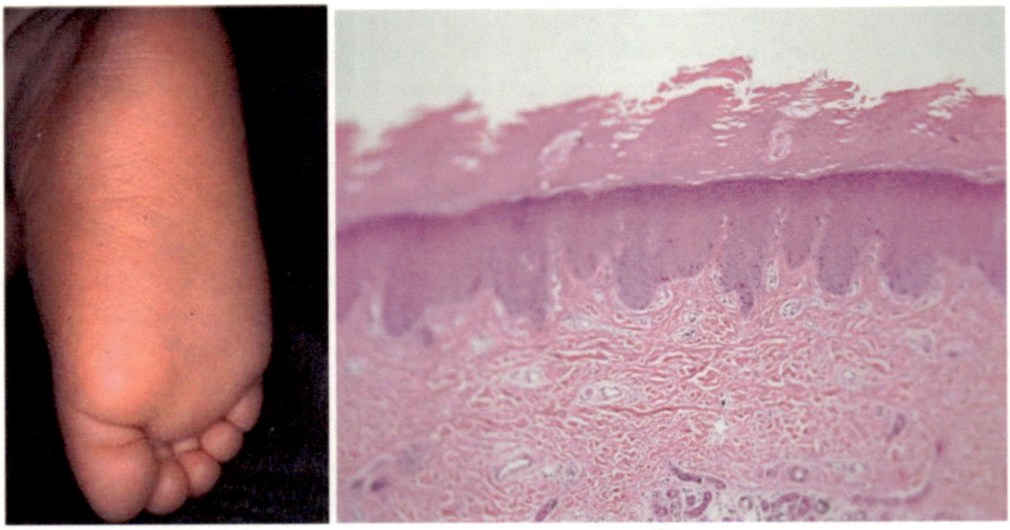

(a) (b)

A 10-month-old Japanese girl presented with bilateral reddish, palmoplantar hyperkeratotic lesions on her palms and soles. The patient was otherwise healthy.

(A) Right sole

(B) Histopathological findings reveal orthokeratotic hyperkeratosis, hypergranulosis, acanthosis, and a mild lymphocytic infiltrate in the upper dermis of the palm.

Figure 1. Nagashima-type PPK

Histological findings include hyperkeratosis, acanthosis, and a thickened granular cell layer with retained nuclei in the stratum corneum. Molecular biology studies have confirmed that the most common mutation is found in the gene encoding connexin 26. This subtype is associated with hearing loss. In contrast, a mutation in the gene for loricrin is associated with mutilating keratoderma and ichthyosis but not deafness. The mode of inheritance for mutation in the loricrin and connexin 26 genes is autosomal dominant. Treatment includes oral retinoids.

2.6. Bart-Pumphrey syndrome

Bart-Pumphrey syndrome is an autosomal-dominant disorder characterized by knuckle pads, leukonychia, PPK and hearing loss. Onset occurs in infancy. PPK may be diffuse and striate, with accentuation of crease patterns and with a grainy surface [5]. Clinically, all neonates are hearing impaired from birth and develop diffuse PPK in childhood. Leukonychia and hyperkeratoses over the joints of the hand may also appear.

Knuckle pads are circumscribed, with hyperkeratotic or fibrous growths over the dorsal aspects of the small joints of the hands or feet. Leukonychia that may be seen in Bart-

Pumphrey syndrome is defined as whiteness of nails that can occur either in patches or involving the total nail. Large keratohyaline granules are found in the keratinocytes, and the keratohyaline-containing cells reflected light, resulting in a white nail appearence. Molecular biology studies reveal a new mutation in the gene that encodes connexin 26, which explains the clinical overlap with Vohwinkel syndrome.

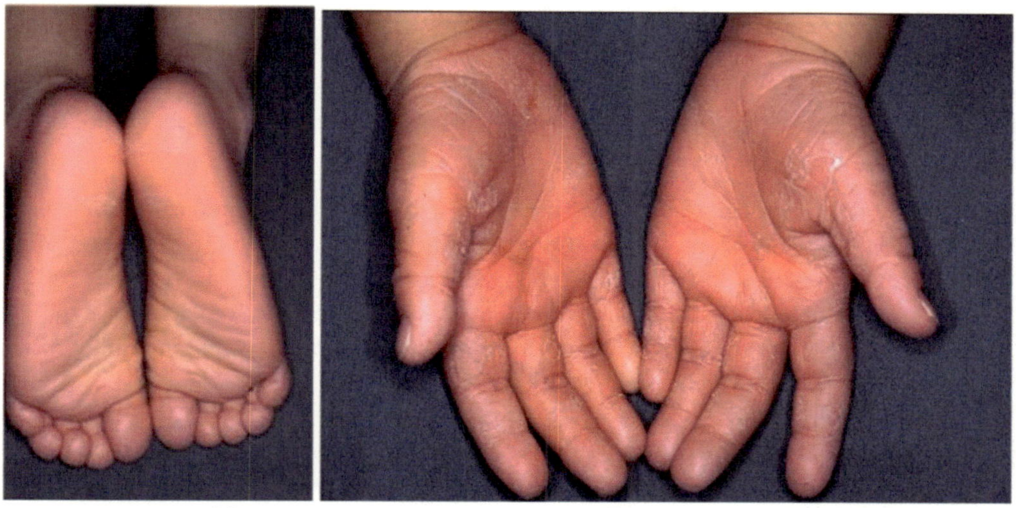

(a) (b)

The patient's sister, a 3-year-old girl, had bilateral reddish palmoplantar hyperkeratotic lesions on the (A) soles and (B) palms. This family had no other significant medical history.

Figure 2. Nagashima-type PPK

2.7. Loricrin keratoderma

The term "loricrin keratoderma" has been suggested to group patients with dominantly inherited PPK that has a different clinical presentation characterized by non-bullous congenital ichthyosiform erythroderma, progressive symmetric erythrokeratoderma, and the patients with Vohwinkel syndrome, carrying mutations in loricrin gene [6, 7]. In all loricrin keratoderma patients, the common signs are the palmoplantar honeycomb hyperkeratosis and ichthyosis. Collodion baby was sometimes reported independently from the clinical evolution of the patients. The originally described Vohwinkel syndrome, because of mutations in connexin 26 gene, shows: palmoplantar honeycomb hyperkeratosis; constricting fibrous bands encircling fingers or toes, characterized as pseudoainhum, leading to autoamputation of the fifth finger due to circulatory impairment; starfish-shaped hyperkeratotic lesions on the extensor surfaces; and high-tone deafness. By contrast, in loricrin keratoderma, the hearing impairment and starfish-shaped hyperkeratosis are absent and a generalized non-erythrodermic ichthyosis is described.

2.8. Clouston syndrome (Hidrotic ectodermal dysplasia)

Clouston syndrome (hidrotic ectodermal dysplasia) is an autosomal dominant ectodermal dysplasia characterized by hypotrichosis, severe nail dystrophy, and PPK as well as hyperpigmentation of the skin over the large joints. Clinical features include diffuse papillomatous PPK (especially over pressure points of the palms and soles), dystrophic nails, and hypotrichosis. Thickened, hyperpigmented skin may also appear over the small and large joints, including the knuckles, elbows, and knees. Thickened, severely dystrophic nails develop, but they may be normal at birth. Universal sparsity of hair involves the scalp, eyebrows, eyelashes, and axillary and genital regions. Sensorineural deafness, polydactyly, syndactyly, clubbing of the fingers, mental retardation, dwarfism, photophobia, and strabismus are associated manifestations.

Clouston syndrome reveals orthohyperkeratosis with a normal granular layer based on histopathological analysis of PPK. Ultrastructural studies of the hair of these patients demonstrate disorganization of hair fibrils with loss of the cuticular cortex. Positional cloning identifies GJB6 on chromosome 13q12 as the causative gene for Clouston syndrome [8].1GJB6 encodes connexin 30 (Cx30), which belongs to a family of cell membrane proteins, the connexins, which form gap junctions between neighbouring cells.

2.9. Olmsted syndrome

Olmsted syndrome is an uncommon genetic disorder with symmetrical, diffuse, transgredient, mutilating PPK and periorificial hyperkeratosis [9]. Most cases of this condition are sporadic, with the exception of one report of an autosomal dominant pattern of inheritance. Onset occurs in the first year of life. Clinically, PPK begins focally in infancy and then becomes diffuse and severe. Later findings include flexion deformities and constriction of the digits, sometimes leading to spontaneous amputation. Progressive, well-defined perioral, perianal, and perineal hyperkeratotic plaques are present, as is onychodystrophy. Alopecia, deafness, nail dystrophy, and dental loss may be associated. Squamous cell carcinoma and malignant melanoma are also known to develop in the affected areas. Rare findings include large joint laxity, ichthyotic lesions, absent premolar teeth, hearing loss for high frequencies, and sclerosing cholangitis.

Histological findings include hyperkeratosis without parakeratosis and mild acanthosis. Abnormal expression of keratin 5 and 14 has been reported. Treatment includes oral and topical retinoids. Full-thickness excision and skin grafting has also been reported to result in clinical improvement.

2.10. Huriez syndrome

Huriez syndrome is an autosomal dominant genodermatosis, characterized by the triad of congenital scleroatrophy of the distal extremities, PPK, and hypoplastic nail changes. The soles are not commonly involved. It was first described in two large pedigrees from northern France [10]. In addition to its occurrence in French patients, it has also been reported in Tunisia, Germany and Italy [11]. Onset occurs in infancy. Clinical features include red, atrophic skin on the dorsal hands and feet at birth. Diffuse, mild keratoderma is more marked on the palms than the soles. Other clinical features are sclerodactyly and nail abnormalities (hypoplasia, fissuring, ridging, koilonychia). The age at the onset of skin cancer is much lower than in the general population, and tumors arise in the areas of the affected skin. Affected individuals carry a more than 100-fold higher risk for the development of aggressive squamous cell carcinoma of the skin.

Histological findings include acanthosis, accentuation of the granular layer, and orthokeratosis. Langerhans cells are almost completely absent in the affected skin. Electron microscopy reveals normal dermoepidermal junctions and desmosomes; however, dense bundles of tonofilaments are seen in the epidermal layer. The granular layer shows large, coarse, clumped keratohyalin. Molecular biology findings include a mutation in the gene mapped to 4q23.

2.11. Papillon-Lefèvre syndrome

Papillon-Lefèvre syndrome is a rare disease characterized by skin lesions, which include PPK and hyperhidrosis with severe periodontal destruction involving both the primary and the permanent dentitions [12]. It is transmitted as an autosomal-recessive condition, and consanguinity of parents is evident in about one-third of the cases. This disease usually has its onset between the ages of 1 to 4 years. The male to female ratio is roughly equal. Its prevalence is estimated to be 1 to 4 per million in the general population with a carrier rate of 2 to 4 per 1000.

Clinically, diffuse transgredient PPK may be observed, typically developing within the first 3 years of life. Punctiform accentuation, particularly along the palmoplantar creases, may be seen. Unless treated, periodontosis results in severe gingivitis and loss of teeth by age 5 years. No significant correlation has been demonstrated between the level of periodontal infection and the severity of skin affections, which supports the concept that these major components of this syndrome are unrelated to each other. Patients exhibit increased susceptibility to cutaneous and systemic infections. Scaly, psoriasiform lesions are often observed over the knees, elbows, and interphalangeal joints. Finally, patients may have malodorous hyperhidrosis.

Histological findings include hyperkeratosis with irregular parakeratosis and moderate perivascular infiltration. Electron microscopic features include lipid-like vacuoles in corneocytes and granulocytes, a reduction in tonofilaments, and irregular keratohyalin granules. Molecular biology findings include mutations in the gene for cathepsin C, mapping to 11q14-q21, which are responsible for this syndrome. Cathepsin C is a lysosomal protease known to activate enzymes that are vital to the body's defenses. The susceptibility factor may involve defective immune function or pleiotropic effect of the single mutant Cathepsin C gene [13].

Treatment includes oral retinoids for the PPK. Elective extraction of involved teeth may prevent excess bone resorption. Appropriate antibiotic therapy may be required for periodontitis and recurrent cutaneous and systemic infections. Treatment with acitretin starting at an early age shows promise in allowing patients to have normal adult dentition. Early treatment and compliance with the prevention program are the major determinants for preserving permanent teeth in young patients. By extracting all primary teeth and eradicating periodontal pathogens, the patient's adult teeth can erupt into a safe environment. Treatment may be more beneficial if it is started during the eruption and maintained during the development of the permanent teeth. Recommended therapy includes aggressive local measures to control plaque including rigorous oral hygiene, chlorhexidine mouth rinses, frequent professional prophylaxis, and periodic appropriate antibiotic therapy needed for long-term maintenance.

2.12. Naxos disease

Naxos disease is a rare autosomal recessive inherited association of right ventricular dysplasia/dilated cardiomyopathy with woolly hair and PPK [14]. The disease has an adverse prognosis, especially in young patients. In a long-term study of an unselected population of patients with Naxos disease it was shown that risk factors for sudden death include history of syncope, the appearance of symptoms, severely progressive disease of the right ventricle before the age of 35 years, and the involvement of the left ventricle [15]. Symptoms of right heart failure appear during the end stages of the disease. One-third of patients become symptomatic before the 30th year of life. In some cases, a few clinical findings of early heart disease can be detected during childhood.

Clinically, a diffuse, nontransgredient keratoderma with an erythematous border appears during the first year of life. Woolly (dense, rough, and bristly) scalp hair is present at birth. Cardiac disease, manifested by arrhythmias, heart failure, or sudden death, becomes evident during and after late puberty. Other cutaneous manifestations include acanthosis nigricans, xerosis, follicular hyperkeratosis over the zygoma, and hyperhidrosis. In addition to the woolly hair at birth, PPK develops during the first year of life and cardiomyopathy is clinically manifested by adolescence with 100% penetrance. Patients present with syncope, sustained ventricular tachycardia or sudden death.

Histological findings include hyperkeratosis, hypergranulosis, and acanthosis. Molecular biology findings include a mutation in the plakoglobin gene, mapping to 17q21, which is responsible for Naxos disease. Plakoglobin is an important component of cell-to-cell and cell-to-matrix adhesion complexes of many tissues, including the skin and cardiac junctions. It also plays a role in signaling in the formation of desmosomal junctions. Mutations in the plakoglobin gene may lead to detachment of the cardiac myocytes, resulting in myocyte death. Plakoglobin mutations may also lead to desmosomal junction fragility in hair shafts, explaining the clinical phenotype of woolly hair.

The primary goal of treatment is the prevention of sudden cardiac death. Implantation of an automatic cardioverter defibrillator is indicated in patients who develop symptoms and/or structural progression, particularly before the age of 35 years. Antiarrhythmic drugs are indicated for preventing recurrence of episodes of sustained ventricular tachycardia. In an attempt to control Naxos disease, systematic genetic screening of the populations at risk has been initiated and is starting to identify the heterozygous carriers of the plakoglobin gene mutation.

3. Focal type

The focal type is subclassified into focal PPK, focal palmoplantar and gingival keratosis, focal keratoderma with oral leukokeratosis, pachyonychia congenita type 1 (Jadassohn–Lawandowsky type) and type 2 (Jackson–Lawler type), and focal PPK associated with esophageal carcinoma. Focal palmoplantar and gingival keratosis is characterized clinically by focal PPK with leukoplakic appearance on the labial surface of the attached gingival lesion, and histologically by focal epidermolytic PPK [16].

4. Striate type

4.1. Striate PPK (Brunauer-Fohs-Siemens syndrome)

Striate PPK (Brunauer-Fohs-Siemens syndrome) presents with linear hyperkeratosis on the palms and fingers and focal plaques on the plantar aspects of the feet. Onset occurs in infancy or the first few years of life. Striate PPK, woolly hair, and left ventricular dilated cardiomyopathy has been described in both autosomal dominant and autosomal recessive forms, but only the recessive forms have a clear association with dilated cardiomyopathy.

Histopathological features include hyperkeratosis, hypergranulosis, and acanthosis with no epidermolysis. Electron microscopic examination shows diminished desmosomes, clumped keratin filaments, and enlarged keratohyalin granules. The syndrome has been linked to mutations in desmoglein 1, desmoplakin, and keratin 1. Treatment may include keratolytics, oral retinoids, and surgical debridement. Striate PPK is known to be caused by heterozygous mutations in either the desmoglein 1 (type I striate PPK), desmoplakin (type II striate PPK) or keratin 1 (type III striate PPK) gene [17-20].

5. Punctate type

5.1. Buschke-Fischer syndrome

Buschke-Fischer syndrome is an autosomal dominant disorder characterized by multiple punctate keratoses over the entire palmoplantar surfaces [21]. Punctate PPK presents as asymptomatic, tiny, hyperkeratotic punctate papules on the palmoplantar surface. Many tiny "raindrop" keratoses involve the palmoplantar surface; skin lesions may involve the whole palmoplantar surface, or may be more restricted in their distribution. The prevalence is 1.17 cases per 100,000 population. The age of onset ranges between 12 and 30 years.

This condition is usually manifested bilaterally as asymptomatic, tiny, hyperkeratotic punctate papules/plaque on the palmoplantar surface. The exact etiology of this disorder is not known, but a dual influence of genetic and environmental factors may trigger the disease. Nail abnormalities in the form of longitudinal ridging, onychorrhexis, onychoschizia, trachyonychia, and notching can be seen. Clinically, asymptomatic, tiny, hyperkeratotic papules are present on the palmoplantar surface. Lesions are uncommon in childhood and usually manifest after age 20 years. This condition is not associated with hyperhidrosis. Patients commonly report pruritus. Most individuals lack associated features; however, spastic paralysis, ankylosing spondylitis, and facial sebaceous hyperplasia have been reported. An association with gastrointestinal and pulmonary malignancy is possible.

Histological findings include substantial compact hyperkeratosis over a distinct area of epidermis, hypergranulosis, the presence of a cornoid lamella, and the absence of epidermal dyskeratosis or hydropic change, which help differentiate this condition from porokeratosis. Two punctate PPK loci have been found to map to 15q22-15q24 and to 8q24.13-8q24.21 [22, 23]. Treatment includes keratolytics, topical salicylic acid, mechanical debridement, excision, and topical and systemic retinoids.

6. Remarks

Hereditary PPK constitutes a heterogeneous group of disorders characterized by thickening of the palms and the soles of individuals who are affected. The diagnosis and classification are difficult due to inter-individual and intra-individual variations and differences in nomenclature. Dermatologists must be alert during the evaluation of these findings to ensure proper diagnosis, and must perform complete dermatological examination including nails, hair, and mucosa. In addition, future studies should include either a whole genome mapping plan or focus directly on candidate genes, such as SLURP1 gene for differential diagnosis between Mal de Meleda and Nagashima-type PPK. More reports and concise clinical observations with genetic approach may reveal the pathomechanism underlying PPK.

Author details

Tamihiro Kawakami
Department of Dermatology, St. Marianna University School of Medicine, Japan

7. References

[1] Lucker GP, Van de Kerkhof PC, Steijlen PM. The hereditary palmoplantar keratoses: an updated review and classification. British Journal of Dermatology 1994;131(1):1-14.

[2] Hamm H, Happle R, Butterfass T, Traupe H. Epidermolytic palmoplantar keratoderma of Vörner: is it the most frequent type of hereditary palmoplantar keratoderma? Dermatologica 1988;177(3):138-145.

[3] Kabashima K, Sakabe J, Yamada Y, Tokura Y. 'Nagashima-type' keratosis as a novel entity in the palmoplantar keratoderma category. Archives of Dermatology 2008;144(3):375-379.

[4] Castro PJS, Fernandez CN, Subirana PQ, Ortiz MP. Vohwinkel Syndrome secondary to missense mutation D66H in GJB2 gene (connexin 26) can include epileptic manifestations. Seizure2010;19(2):129-131.

[5] Ramer JC, Vasily DB, Ladda RL. Familial leukonychia, knuckle pads, hearing loss, and palmoplantar hyperkeratosis: An additional family with Bart-Pumphrey syndrome. Journal of Medical Genetics 1994;31(1):68-71.

[6] Ishida-Yamamoto A, McGrath JA, Lam H, Iizuka H, Friedman RA, Christiano AM. The molecular pathology of progressive symmetric erythrokeratoderma: a frameshift mutation in the loricrin gene and perturbations in the cornified cell envelope. American Journal of Human Genetics 1997;61(3):581-589.

[7] Ishida-Yamamoto A. Loricrin keratoderma: a novel disease entity characterized by nuclear accumulation of mutant loricrin. Journal of Dermatological Science 2003;31(1):3-8.

[8] Lamartine J, Munhoz Essenfelder G, Kibar Z, Lanneluc I, Callouet E, Laoudj D, Lemaître G, Hand C, Hayflick SJ, Zonana J, Antonarakis S, Radhakrishna U, Kelsell DP, Christianson AL, Pitaval A, Der Kaloustian V, Fraser C, Blanchet-Bardon C, Rouleau GA, Waksman G. Mutations in GJB6 cause hidrotic ectodermal dysplasia. Nature Genetics 2000;26(2):142-144.

[9] Bergonse FN, Rabello SM, Barreto RL, Romiti R, Nico MM, Aoki V, Reis VM, Rivitti EA. Olmsted syndrome: The clinical spectrum of mutilating palmoplantar keratoderma. Pediatric Dermatology 2003;20(4):323-326.

[10] Huriez C, Deminatti M, Agache P, Mennecier M. A gene dysplasia not previously known: frequently degenerative sclero-atrophying and keratodermic genodermatosis of the extremities. Sem Hop journal 1968;44(8):481-488.

[11] Watanabe E, Takai T, Ichihashi M, Ueda M. A Non familial Japanese case of Huriez syndrome:p 53 expression in squamous cell carcinoma. Dermatology 2003;207(1):82-84.

[12] Angel TA, Hsu S, Kornbleuth SI, Kornbleuth J, Kramer EM. Papillon-Lefèvre syndrome: A case report of four affected siblings. Journal of the American Academy of Dermatology 2002;46(2 Suppl):S8-S10.

[13] Hart TC, Hart PS, Michalec MD, Zhang Y, Marazita ML, Cooper M, Yassin OM, Nusier M, Walker S. Localization of a gene for prepubertal periodontitis to chromosome 11q14 and identification of a cathepsin C gene mutation. Journal of Medical Genetics 2000;37(2):95-101.

[14] Protonotarios N, Tsatsopoulou A, Patsourakos P, Alexopoulos D, Gezerlis P, Simitsis S, Scampardonis G. Cardiac abnormalities in familial palmoplantar keratosis. British Heart Journal 1986;56(4):321-326.

[15] Protonotarios N, Tsatsopoulou A, Anastasakis A, Sevdalis E, McKoy G, Stratos K, Gatzoulis K, Tentolouris K, Spiliopoulou C, Panagiotakos D, McKenna W, Toutouzas P. Genotype-phenotype assessment in autosomal recessive arrhythmogenic right ventricular cardiomyopathy (Naxos disease) caused by a deletion in plakoglobin. Journal of the American College of Cardiology 2001;38(5):1477-1484.

[16] Kolde G, Hennies HC, Bethke G, Reichart PA. Focal palmoplantar and gingival keratosis: a distinct palmoplantar ectodermal dysplasia with epidermolytic alternations

but lack of mutations in known keratins. Journal of the American Academy of Dermatology 2005;52(3 Pt 1):403-409.

[17] Armstrong DK, McKenna KE, Purkis PE, Green KJ, Eady RA, Leigh IM, Hughes AE. Haploinsufficiency of desmoplakin causes a striate subtype of palmoplantar keratoderma. Human Molecular Genetics 1988;8(1):143-148.

[18] Whittock NV, Ashton GH, Dopping-Hepenstal PJ, Gratian MJ, Keane FM, Eady RA, McGrath JA. Striate palmoplantar keratoderma resulting from desmoplakin haploinsufficiency. Journal of Investigative Dermatology 1999;113(6):940-946.

[19] Hunt DM, Rickman L, Whittock NV, Eady RA, Simrak D, Dopping-Hepenstal PJ, Stevens HP, Armstrong DK, Hennies HC, Küster W, Hughes AE, Arnemann J, Leigh IM, McGrath JA, Kelsell DP, Buxton RS. Spectrum of dominant mutations in the desmosomal cadherin desmoglein 1, causing the skin disease striate palmoplantar keratoderma. European Journal of Human Genetics 2001;9(3):197-203.

[20] Whittock NV, Smith FJ, Wan H, Mallipeddi R, Griffiths WA, Dopping-Hepenstal P, Ashton GH, Eady RA, McLean WH, McGrath JA. Frameshift mutation in the V2 domain of human keratin 1 results in striate palmoplantar keratoderma. Journal of Investigative Dermatology 2002;118(5):838-844.

[21] Oztas P, Alli N, Polat M, Dagdelen S, Ustün H, Artüz F, Erdemli E. Punctate palmoplantar keratoderma (Brauer-Buschke-Fischer syndrome). American Journal of Clinical Dermatology 2007;8(2):113-116.

[22] Martinez-Mir A, Zlotogorski A, Londono D, Gordon D, Grunn A, Uribe E, Horev L, Ruiz IM, Davalos NO, Alayan O, Liu J, Gilliam TC, Salas-Alanis JC, Christiano AM. Identification of a locus for type I punctate palmoplantar keratoderma on chromosome 15q22–q24. Journal of Medical Genetics 2003;40(12):872-878.

[23] Zhang XJ, Li M, Gao TW, He PP, Wei SC, Liu JB, Li CR, Cui Y, Yang S, Yuan WT, Li CY, Liu YF, Xu SJ, Huang W. Identification of a locus for punctate palmoplantar keratodermas at chromosome 8q24.13–8q24.21. Journal of Investigative Dermatology 2004;122(5):1121-1125.

Chapter 5

LEKTI: Netherton Syndrome and Atopic Dermatitis

Naoki Oiso and Akira Kawada

Additional information is available at the end of the chapter

http://dx.doi.org/10.5772/53574

1. Introduction

Netherton syndrome is an uncommon autosomal recessive disorder characterized by congenital ichthyosis with defective cornification, bamboo hair, and severe atopic manifestation. It is caused by mutations in *SPINK5*. Atopic dermatitis is shown to be associated with polymorphisms in *SPINK5*.

In 1958, Netherton described the bamboo-like deformity in the fragile hairs in a girl with erythematous scaly dermatitis.[2] In 1985, Greene and Muller emphasized the triad of Netherton syndrome: ichthyosis, atopy, and trichorrhexis invaginata.[3] In 2000, Chavanas *et al.* identified eleven different mutations in *SPINK5* in 13 families with Netherton syndrome.[4] Their finding disclosed a critical role of the serine protease inhibitor lymphoepithelial Kazal-type related inhibitor (LEKTI) in epidermal barrier function and immunity, suggesting a sequential pathway for high serum IgE levels and atopic manifestations.[4] In 2005, Descargues *et al.* found that LEKTI is a key regulator of epidermal protease activity and degradation of desmoglein 1 as the primary pathogenic event.[5] In 2010, Sales showed that a pathogenic matriptase-pro-kallikrein pathway could operate in a variety of physiological and pathological processes.[6] Thus, the study of Netherton syndrome contributes not only elucidation of pathogenesis of the disorder itself but also understanding of structure of the epidermis and immune and inflammatory processes including atopic dermatitis.

In this session, we summarize (1) the clinical features of Netherton syndrome, (2) the genetic relationship of *SPINK5* to atopic dermatitis, and (3) the molecular functions.

2. The clinical features of Netherton syndrome

Netherton syndrome is an uncommon autosomal recessive disease characterized by ichthyosis linearis circumflexa and/or congenital ichthyosiform erythroderma, hair shaft defects including trichorrhexis invaginata, trichorrhexis nodosa and pili torti and atopic manifestations with an elevated IgE level, frequent asthma and food allergies.[1] It is caused by mutations in *SPINK5* encoding LEKTI.

The infants with Netherton syndrome commonly show a generalized erythroderma covered by fine, translucent scales, which can be difficult to distinguish clinically from erythrodermic psoriasis, non-bullous congenital ichthyosiform erythroderma, or other infantile erythrodermas.[7] Electron microscopy is useful for diagnosis. It illustrates premature lamellar body secretions and foci of electron-dense materials in the intercellular spaces of stratum corneum.[7] Patients with a mild phenotype of ichthyosis linearis circumflexa on the palms and soles will have mutations located downstream near the C-terminal end, while a severe erythrodermic phenotype will be associated with nucleotide changes with early truncations in *SPINK5*.[8, 9]

Trichorrhexis invaginata (bamboo hair) is a focal defect of the hair shaft that produces development of torsion nodules and invaginated nodules.[1] Invagination of affected hairs is caused by softness of the cortex in the keratogenous zone because of an incomplete formation of disulfide bonds.[10]

Lack of LEKTI causes stratum corneum detachment secondary to epidermal proteases hyperactivity.[11] This skin barrier defect favors allergen absorption and is generally regarded as the underlying cause for atopic dermatitis-like lesions in Netherton syndrome.[11] Uncontrolled kallikreins (KLK)s activity in Netherton syndrome epidermis can trigger atopic dermatitis-like lesions, independently of the environment and the adaptive immune system.[11]

3. The genetic relationship of *SPINK5* to atopic dermatitis

Atopic dermatitis is a chronic and relapsing inflammatory skin disorder caused by multiple genetic and environmental factors. A recent genome-wide association studies for atopic dermatitis identified susceptibility loci at 1q21.3 (*FLG*), 5q22.1 (*TMEM232* and *SLC25A46*) and 20q13.33 (*TNFRSF6B* and *ZGPAT*) in the Chinese samples (4,636 cases and 13,559 controls),[12] and a genome-wide association meta-analysis detected susceptibility loci at 11q13.5 (*OVOL1*), 19p13.2 (*ACTL9*), and 5q22.1 (*KIF3A*) in 5,606 affected individuals and 20,565 controls from 16 population-based cohorts and an additional 5,419 affected individuals and 19,833 controls from 14 studies.[13] Andiappan *et al.* showed no evidence of association of the locus at 5q22.1, even though the effect sizes in the Singaporean Chinese population are similar to that reported in Sun *et al.*[12, 14] These results indicate that atopic dermatitis is more multi-factors-involved and complicated disorder than vitiligo and alopecia areata.[15, 16]

Association of *SPINK5* gene polymorphisms with atopic dermatitis has been shown in case-control studies,[17-20] even though genome-wide association studies for atopic dermatisis have not identified the statistic significance. It would be indispensable to accumulate patients with typical atopic dramatis, which should be classified into the extrinsic or intrinsic types, and distinct healthy controls with no family and personal history of atopic dermatitis, allergic rhinitis and/or asthma for next investigation of genome-wide association studies for atopic dermatitis.

Fortugno *et al.* investigated the functional difference between representative associated polymorphism, Glu420Lys, because glutamic acid (Glu E) is an acidic amino acid and lysine (Lys K) is a basic.[21] They showed increased epidermal protease activity correlates with reduced desmoglein 1 protein expression and accelerated profilaggrin proteolysis under the presence of residue 420K within the *SPINK5* sequence, contributing to defective skin barrier permeability.[21] They found that epidermis with homozygous lysine residues in codon 420 in *SPINK5* displays an increased expression of the proallergic cytokine thymic stromal lymphopoietin (TSLP).[21] Further functional analysis would shed light on the involvement of the decreased activity of LEKTI in atopic dermatitis.

4. The molecular functions

The epidermis consists of the basal layer, the spinous layer, the granular layer and the cornified layer. The hair follicle is constructed by the inner root sheath, the outer root sheath and the hair bulb. LEKTI is expressed in the granular layer of the epidermis and in the inner root sheet of hair follicle and acts as an inhibitor of multiple serine proteases. [4] LEPTI contains fifteen serine protease inhibitor domains and its proteolytic fragments inhibit epidermal proteases. [22-28] LEPTI can inhibit the epidermal serine protease KLK5, KLK6, KLK7, KLK13 and KLK14. [29] LEKTI-domain 6 was shown to specifically inhibit KLK5 and KLK7 in the mid-to-high nanomolar range. [30] Thus, protease inhibitors such as LEPTI are crucial players for controlling protease activity.

KLK5 can cleave desmoglein 1, inducing the detachment of stratum corneum and subsequent severe skin barrier defect which is associated with high permeability of various allergens. Unrepressed KLK5 activity can be present in loss-of-functional mutation in *SPINK5* in Netherton syndrome and decreased functional polymorphisms in *SPINK5* in atopic dermatitis. Unrestrained KLK5 activates an autonomous protease-activated-receptor-2 (PAR2) signaling, resulting in the production of major-pro-inflammatory molecules and pro-T helper 2 cytokines such as TSLP.[31] The specific KLK5-PAR-2-TSLP pathway induces atopic dermatitis-like lesions in Netherton syndrome and atopic dermatitis in individuals with predisposed polymorphisms.

KLK7 is involved in stratum corneum desquamation via the disruption of corneodesmosomes and the cell-cell adhesion junctions of corneocytes by hydrolyzing the two mayor cadherins (corneodesmosin and desmocollin 1) in the extracellular region of the junctions. [32]

Matriptase is a transmembrane tripsin-like serine protease having the capacity of autoactivation and subsequent occurrence of proteolytic cascade reactions.[33, 34] Sales *et al.* showed that matriptase is an efficient activator of epidermal pro-KLKs that co-localize with LEKTI at the granular-transitional layer boundary where epidermal separation takes place in Netherton syndrome.[6] They demonstrated that all the central manifestations of Netherton syndrome in LEKTI-deficient mice, such as aberrant proteolytic activity in the lower epidermis, corneodesmosome fragility, stratum corneum loss and skin inflammation, depend on the epidermal expression of matriptase.[6] Thus, pro-KLKs might be activated as KLKs which trigger excess proteolytic function under the functional loss of LEKTI in Netherton syndrome or functional insufficiency of LEKTI in atopic dermatitis with decreased functional polymorphisms in *SPINK5*.

The functional loss or insufficiency of LEKTI induces relative excess activation of serine protease toward severe skin allergy.

5. Conclusion

Recently, studies for the interaction between proteases and protease inhibitors are focused on the elucidation of pathogenesis of Netherton syndrome, atopic dermatitis, asthma, and food allergies. Atopic manifestation with an elevated IgE level in Netherton syndrome prompted researches to investigate the genetic relationship between atopic dermatitis and genetic polymorphisms. LEKTI encoded by functionally decreased polymorphisms can alter proteolytic activation and protease deregulation. The relationship between atopic dermatitis and improper cornification has been focused not only in model mice of Netherton syndrome but also in flaky tail mice with double filaggrin and loricrin deficiencies.[35] Further study will discover more precise mechanism in cornification, which would provide novel strategies for effective treatment for Netherton syndrome and atopic dermatitis.

Author details

Naoki Oiso and Akira Kawada
Departments of Dermatology, Kinki University Faculty of Medicine, Osaka-Sayama, Osaka, Japan

6. References

[1] Sun JD, Linden KG. Netherton syndrome: successful use of topical tacrolimus and pimecrolimus in four siblings. Int J Dermatol 2006; 45: 693-7.
[2] Netherton EW. A unique case of trichorrhexis nodosa; bamboo hairs. AMA Arch Derm 1958; 78: 483-7.
[3] Greene SL, Muller SA. Netherton's syndrome. Report of a case and review of the literature. J Am Acad Dermatol 1985; 13: 329-37.
[4] Chavanas S, Bodemer C, Rochat A, *et al.* Mutations in SPINK5, encoding a serine protease inhibitor, cause Netherton syndrome. Nat Genet 2000; 25: 141-2.
[5] Descargues P, Deraison C, Bonnart C, *et al.* Spink5-deficient mice mimic Netherton syndrome through degradation of desmoglein 1 by epidermal protease hyperactivity. Nat Genet 2005; 37: 56-65.

[6] Sales KU, Masedunskas A, Bey AL, *et al*. Matriptase initiates activation of epidermal pro-kallikrein and disease onset in a mouse model of Netherton syndrome. Nat Genet 2010; 42: 676-83.
[7] Fartasch M, Williams ML, Elias PM, *et al*. Altered lamellar body secretion and stratum corneum membrane structure in Netherton syndrome: differentiation from other infantile erythrodermas and pathogenic implications. *Arch Dermatol* 1999; 135: 823-32.
[8] Sprecher E, Chavanas S, DiGiovanna JJ *et al*. The spectrum of pathogenic mutations in SPINK5 in 19 families with Netherton syndrome: implications for mutation detection and first case of prenatal diagnosis. J Invest Dermatol 2001; 117: 179-87.
[9] Mizuno Y, Suga Y, Muramatsu S, *et al*. A Japanese infant with localized ichthyosis linearis circumflexa on the palms and soles harbouring a compound heterozygous mutation in the SPINK5 gene. Br J Dermatol 2005; 153: 661-3.
[10] Ito M, Ito K, Hashimoto K. Pathogenesis in trichorrhexis invaginata (bamboo hair). *J Invest Dermatol* 1984; 83: 1-6.
[11] Briot A, Deraison C, Lacroix M, *et al*. Kallikrein 5 induces atopic dermatitis-like lesions through PAR2-mediated thymic stromal lymphopoietin expression in Netherton syndrome. J Exp Med 2009; 206: 1135-47.
[12] Sun LD, Xiao FL, Li Y, *et al*. Genome-wide association study identifies two new susceptibility loci for atopic dermatitis in the Chinese Han population. Nat Genet 2011; 43: 690-4.
[13] Paternoster L, Standl M, Chen CM, *et al*. Meta-analysis of genome-wide association studies identifies three new risk loci for atopic dermatitis. Nat Genet 2011; 44: 187-92.
[14] Andiappan AK, Foo JN, Choy MW, *et al*. Validation of GWAS loci for atopic dermatitis in a Singapore Chinese population. J Invest Dermatol 2012; 132: 1505-7.
[15] Jin Y, Birlea SA, Fain PR, *et al*. Genome-wide association analyses identify 13 new susceptibility loci for generalized vitiligo. Nat Genet 2012; 44: 676-80.
[16] Petukhova L, Duvic M, Hordinsky M, *et al*. Genome-wide association study in alopecia areata implicates both innate and adaptive immunity. Nature 2010; 466: 113-7.
[17] Walley AJ, Chavanas S, Moffatt MF, *et al*. Gene polymorphism in Netherton and common atopic disease. Nat Genet 2001; 29: 175-8.
[18] Kato A, Fukai K, Oiso N, *et al*. Association of SPINK5 gene polymorphisms with atopic dermatitis in the Japanese population. Br J Dermatol 2003; 148: 665-9.
[19] Lan CC, Tu HP, Wu CS, *et al*. Distinct SPINK5 and IL-31 polymorphisms are associated with atopic eczema and non-atopic hand dermatitis in Taiwanese nursing population. Exp Dermatol 2011; 20: 975-9.
[20] Zhao LP, Di Z, Zhang L, *et al*. Association of SPINK5 gene polymorphisms with atopic dermatitis in Northeast China. J Eur Acad Dermatol Venereol 2012; 26: 572-7.
[21] Fortugno P, Furio L, Teson M, *et al*. The 420K LEKTI variant alters LEKTI proteolytic activation and results in protease deregulation: implications for atopic dermatitis. Hum Mol Genet, in press.
[22] Bitoun E, Micheloni A, Lamant L *et al*. LEKTI proteolytic processing in human primary keratinocytes, tissue distribution and defective expression in Netherton syndrome. Hum Mol Genet 2003; 12: 2417-30.

[23] Egelrud T, Brattsand M, Kreutzmann P *et al.* hK5 and hK7, two serine proteinases abundant in human skin, are inhibited by LEKTI domain 6. Br J Dermatol 2005; 153: 1200-3.

[24] Borgono CA, Michael IP, Komatsu N *et al.* A potential role for multiple tissue kallikrein serine proteases in epidermal desquamation. J Biol Chem 2007; 282: 3640-52.

[25] Deraison C, Bonnart C, Lopez F *et al.* LEKTI fragments specifically inhibit KLK5, KLK7, and KLK14 and control desquamation through a pH-dependent interaction. Mol Biol Cell 2007; 18: 3607-19.

[26] Ovaere P, Lippens S, Vandenabeele P, *et al.* The emerging roles of serine protease cascades in the epidermis. Trends Biochem Sci 2009; 34: 453-63.

[27] Fortugno P, Bresciani A, Paolini C *et al.* Proteolytic activation cascade of the Netherton Syndrome-Defective Protein, LEKTI, in the epidermis: implications for skin homeostasis. J Invest Dermatol 2011; 131: 2223-32.

[28] Lacroix M, Lacaze-Buzy L, Furio L, *et al.* Clinical expression and new SPINK5 splicing defects in Netherton syndrome: unmasking a frequent founder synonymous mutation and unconventional intronic mutations. J Invest Dermatol 2012; 132: 575-82.

[29] Borgoño CA, Michael IP, Komatsu N, *et al.* A potential role for multiple tissue kallikrein serine proteases in epidermal desquamation. J Biol Chem 2007; 282: 3640-52.

[30] Egelrud T, Brattsand M, Kreutzmann P, *et al.* hK5 and hK7, two serine proteinases abundant in human skin, are inhibited by LEKTI domain 6. *Br J Dermatol* 2005; 153: 1200-3.

[31] Furio L, Hovnanian A. When activity requires breaking up: LEKTI proteolytic activation cascade for specific proteinase inhibition. J Invest Dermatol 2011; 131: 2169-73.

[32] Fernández IS, Ständker L, Mägert HJ, *et al.* Crystal structure of human epidermal kallikrein 7 (hK7) synthesized directly in its native state in E. coli: insights into the atomic basis of its inhibition by LEKTI domain 6 (LD6). J Mol Biol 2008; 377: 1488-97.

[33] Takeuchi T, Harris JL, Huang W, *et al.* Cellular localization of membrane-type serine protease 1 and identification of protease-activated receptor-2 and single-chain urokinase-type plasminogen activator as substrates. J Biol Chem 2000; 275: 26333-42.

[34] Lee SL, Dickson RB, Lin CY. Activation of hepatocyte growth factor and urokinase/plasminogen activator by matriptase, an epithelial membrane serine protease. J Biol Chem 2000; 275: 36720-5.

[35] Nakai K, Yoneda K, Hosokawa Y, *et al.* Reduced expression of epidermal growth factor receptor, e-cadherin, and occludin in the skin of flaky tail mice is due to filaggrin and loricrin deficiencies. Am J Pathol 2012; 181: 969-77.

Chapter 6

Discovery and Delineation of Dermatan 4-*O*-Sulfotransferase-1 (D4ST1)-Deficient Ehlers-Danlos Syndrome

Tomoki Kosho

Additional information is available at the end of the chapter

http://dx.doi.org/10.5772/55026

1. Introduction

The Ehlers-Danlos syndrome (EDS) is a heterogeneous group of heritable connective tissue disorders affecting as many as 1 in 5000 individuals, characterized by joint and skin laxity, and tissue fragility [1]. The fundamental mechanisms of EDS are known to consist of dominant-negative effects or haploinsufficiency of mutant procollagen α-chains and deficiency of collagen-processing-enzymes [2]. In a revised nosology established in the nomenclature conference held in June 1997 at Villefranche-sur-Mer, France, Beighton et al. [3] classified EDS into six major types (Table 1): classical type (OMIM#130000), hypermobility type (OMIM#130020), vascular type (OMIM#130050), kyphoscoliosis type (OMIM#225400), arthrochalasia type (OMIM#130060), and dermatosparaxis type (OMIM#225410). Additional minor variants of EDS have been identified with molecular and biochemical abnormalities: dermatan 4-*O*-sulfotransferase-1 (D4ST1)-deficient type/musculocontractural type (OMIM#601776), Brittle cornea syndrome (OMIM#229200), EDS-like syndrome due to tenascin-XB deficiency (OMIM#606408), EDS with progressive kyphoscoliosis, myopathy, and hearing loss (OMIM#614557); the spondylocheiro dysplastic form (OMIM#612350), cardiac valvular form (OMIM#225320), and progeroid form (OMIM#130070) [4] (Table 1). This chapter focuses on a recent breakthrough in EDS: discovery and delineation of D4ST1-deficient EDS (DD-EDS).

2. History of D4ST1-deficient EDS

DD-EDS, caused by loss-of-function mutations in the carbohydrate sulfotransferase 14 (*CHST14*) gene coding D4ST1, has been identified independently as a rare type of arthrogryposis syndrome, "adducted thumb–clubfoot syndrome (ATCS)" [5]; as a specific form of EDS, "EDS, Kosho Type" (EDSKT) [6]; and as a subset of kyphoscoliosis type EDS without evidence of lysyl hydroxylase deficiency, "Musculocontractural EDS" (MCEDS) [7].

	Prevalence §	Inheritance	Causative gene(s)
Major types			
Classical type	1/20,000	AD	*COL5A1, COL5A2*
Hypermobility type	1/5,000-20,000	AD	*TNXB*#
Vascular type	1/50,000-250,000	AD	*COL3A1*
Kyphoscoliosis type	1/100,000	AR	*PLOD*
Arthrochalacia type	30	AD	*COL1A1**, *COL1A2**
Dermatosparaxis type	8	AR	*ADAMTS-2*
Other variants			
D4ST1-deficient type	26	AR	*CHST14*
Brittle cornea syndrome	11	AR	*ZNF469*
EDS-like syndrome due to tenascin-XB deficiency	10	AR	*TNXB*
EDS with progressive kyphoscoliosis myopathy, and hearing loss	7	AR	*FKBP14*
Spondylocheiro dysplastic form	8	AR	SLC39A13
Cardiac valvular form	4	AR	*COL1A2*
Progeroid form	3	AR	*B4GALT7*

§, a fraction number represents the prevalence such as "one affected person in 20,000 individuals" for "1/20,000" and an integral number represents the sum of previously reported patients; AD, autosomal dominant; AR, autosomal recessive; *COL5A1* or *COL5A2*, α1(V) or α2(V) procollagen; *TNXB*, tenascin-X; #, in a small subset of cases; *COL3A1*, α1(III) procollagen; *PLOD*; lysyl hydroxylase; *COL1A1* or *COL1A2*, α1(I) or α2(I) procollagen; *, splice-site mutations of the genes; *ADAMTS2*; procollagen I N-proteinase; *CHST14*, carbohydrate sulfotransferase 14; *ZNF469*, zinc finger protein 469; *FKBP14*, FK506-binding protein 14; *SLC39A13*, a membrane-bound zinc transporter; *B4GALT7*; xylosylprotein 4-beta-galactosyltransferase

Table 1. Classification of Ehlers-Danlos Syndromes

2.1. Adducted thumb–Clubfoot syndrome

The original report of ATCS was written by Dündar et al. [8] from Erciyes University, Turkey, presenting two cousins, a boy aged 3.5 years and a girl aged 1.5 years, from a consanguineous Turkish family. In common, they had moderate to severe psychomotor developmental delay, ocular anterior chamber abnormality, facial characteristics, generalized joint laxity, arachnodactyly, camptodactyly, and distal arthrogryposis with adducted thumbs and clubfeet. They reported another patient with ATCS, a boy aged 3 months, from a consanguineous Turkish family including three affected siblings who died of unknown etiology between the ages of 1 and 4 months [9]. The patient also had bilateral nephrolithiasis, a unilateral inguinal hernia, and bilateral cryptorchidism. The authors suggested that two brothers, aged 22 months and 7 months, from a Japanese consanguineous family reported by Sonoda and Kouno [10] would also fit the diagnosis of ATCS. The brothers had multiple distal arthrogryposis, characteristic facial features, cleft palates, short stature, hydronephrosis, cryptorchidism, and normal intelligence. Dündar et al. [9] also showed follow-up observations of the original patients: the intelligence quotient (IQ) was roughly 90 in one subject at age 7 years and 2 months and the other died of unknown cause at 5 years of age. Janecke et al. [11] from Innsbruck Medical University, Austria, reported two brothers with ATCS from a consanguineous Austrian family, one of whom died shortly after birth because of respiratory failure. The authors concluded that all these patients represented a new type of arthrogryposis with central nervous system involvement, congenital heart defects, urogenital defects, myopathy, connective tissue involvement (generalized joint laxity), and normal or subnormal mental development. In 2009, Dündar et al. reported that *CHST14* was the causal gene for ATCS through homozygosity mapping using samples from four previously published consanguineous families. The authors mentioned some follow-up clinical findings including generalized joint laxity, delayed wound healing, ecchymoses, hematomas, and osteopenia/osteoporosis; and categorized ATCS as a generalized connective tissue disorder [5].

2.2. EDS, Kosho type

We encountered the first patient with a specific type of EDS in 2000 and the second with parental consanguinity in 2003. They were Japanese girls with strikingly similar symptoms: characteristic craniofacial features; skeletal features including multiple congenital contractures, malfanoid habitus, pectus excavatum, generalized joint laxity, recurrent dislocations, and progressive talipes and spinal deformity; skin hyperextensibility, bruisability, and fragility with atrophic scars; recurrent hematomas; and hypotonia with mild motor developmental delay [12]. These symptoms overlapped those in the kyphoscoliosis type EDS (previously known as EDS type VI), which is typically associated with deficiency of lysyl hydroxylase (EDS type VIA) [13]. A rare condition with the clinical phenotype of the kyphoscoliosis type EDS but with normal lysyl hydroxylase activity were reported and named as EDS type VIB [13]. Therefore, we tentatively proposed that the two patients represented a clinically recognizable subgroup of EDS type VIB [12]. Through their long-term clinical evaluation as well as four additional unrelated Japanese patients including one with parental consanguinity and another reported by Yasui et al. [14], we concluded that they—four female patients and two male patients aged 4–32 years, represented a new clinically recognized type of EDS with distinct craniofacial characteristics, multiple congenital contractures, progressive joint and skin laxity, and multisystem fragility-related manifestations [15]. The disorder has been registered as EDS Kosho Type (EDSKT) in the London Dysmorphology Database (http://www.lmdatabases.com/index.html) and in POSSUM (http://www.possum.net.au/). In 2009, we identified *CHST14* as causal for the disorder through homozygosity mapping using samples from two consanguineous families and all the other patients were also found to have compound heterozygous *CHST14* mutations [6].

2.3. Musculocontractural EDS

Malfait et al. [7] from Ghent University, Belgium have found mutations in *CHST14* through homozygosity mapping of two Turkish sisters and an Indian girl both presenting clinically with EDS VIB and with parental consanguinity. They had distinct craniofacial features, joint contractures, and wrinkled palms in addition to common features of kyphoscoliosis type EDS including kyphoscoliosis, muscular hypotonia, hyperextensible, thin, and bruisable skin, atrophic scarring, joint hypermobility, and variable ocular involvement. Malfait et al. [7] concluded that their series and ATCS, as well as EDSKT, formed a phenotypic continuum based on their clinical observations and identification of an identical mutation in both conditions; and proposed to coin the disorder as "musculocontractural EDS" (MCEDS).

3. Pathophysiology of D4ST1-deficient EDS

3.1. Glycobiological abnormalities in D4ST1-deficient EDS

D4ST1 is a regulatory enzyme in the glycosaminoglycan (GAG) biosynthesis that transfers active sulfate to position 4 of the N-acetyl-D-galactosamine residues of dermatan sulfate (DS) (Fig. 1) [16, 17]. DS, together with chondroitin sulfate (CS) and heparan sulfate, constitutes GAG chains of proteoglycans and is implicated in cardiovascular disease, tumorigenesis, infection, wound repair, and fibrosis via DS-containing proteoglycans such as decorin and biglycan [18].

Sulfotransferase activity toward dermatan in the skin fibroblasts derived from the patients was significantly decreased to 6.7% (patient 1 with a compound heterozygous mutation: P281L/Y293C) and 14.5% (patient 3 with a homozygous mutation: P281L) of each age- and sex-matched control) (Fig. 2A). Disaccharide composition analysis of CS/DS chains isolated from the skin fibroblasts showed a negligible amount of DS and a slight excess of CS (Fig. 2B). Subsequently, we focused on a major DS proteoglycan in the skin, decorin, consisting of core protein and one GAG chain and playing an important role in assembly of collagen fibrils (Nomura, 2006). No DS disaccharides were detected in the GAG chains of decorin from the patients, whereas the GAG chains of decorin from the controls were mainly composed of DS disaccharides (approximately 95%) (Fig. 2C) [6].

3.2. Pathological abnormalities in D4ST1-deficient EDS

Hematoxylin and eosin (H&E)-stained light microscopy on patients' skin specimens showed that fine collagen fibers were present predominantly in the reticular to papillary dermis with marked reduction of normally thick collagen bundles (Fig. 3a, b). Electron microscopy showed that collagen fibrils were dispersed in the reticular dermis, compared with the regularly and tightly assembled ones observed in the control; whereas each collagen fibril was smooth and round, not varying in size and shape, similar to each fibril of the control (Fig. 3c, d) [6].

Patient	Family	Origin	*CHST14* mutations	Sex	Age at initial publication	References
1	1	Turkish	V49X homo	F	3.5y	[8]
2				M	1.5y	
3				F	6y	
4	2	Japanese	Y293C homo	M	4y	[10]
5				M	7m	
6	3	Austrian	R213P homo	M	0d†	[11]
7				M	12m	
8	4	Turkish	[R135G;L137Q] homo	F	1–4m†	[9]
9				M	1–4m†	
10				M	1–4m†	
11				M	3m	
12	5	Japanese	P281L/Y293C	F	11y	[12]
13	6	Japanese	P281L homo	F	14y	[12]
14	7	Japanese	P281L homo	M	32y	[15]
15	8	Japanese	K69X/P281L	M	32y	[14,15]
16	9	Japanese	P281L/C289S	F	20y	[15]
17	10	Japanese	P281L/Y293C	F	4y	[15]
18	11	Turkish	V49X homo	F	22y	[7]
19				F	21y	
20	12	Indian	E334Gfs*107 homo	F	12y	[7]
21	13	Japanese	P281L/Y293C	M	2y	[21]
22	14	Japanese	F209S/P281L	M	6y	[21]
23	15	Dutch	V48X homo	F	20y	[23]
24	16	Afghani	R274P homo	F	11y	[24]
25				F	0y	
26	17	Miccosukee	G228Lfs*13	F	16y	[25]

homo, homozygous mutation; /, compound heterozygous mutation; F, female; M, male; y, years old; m, months old; †, dead at the time of publication

Table 2. Reported patients with D4ST1-deficient EDS

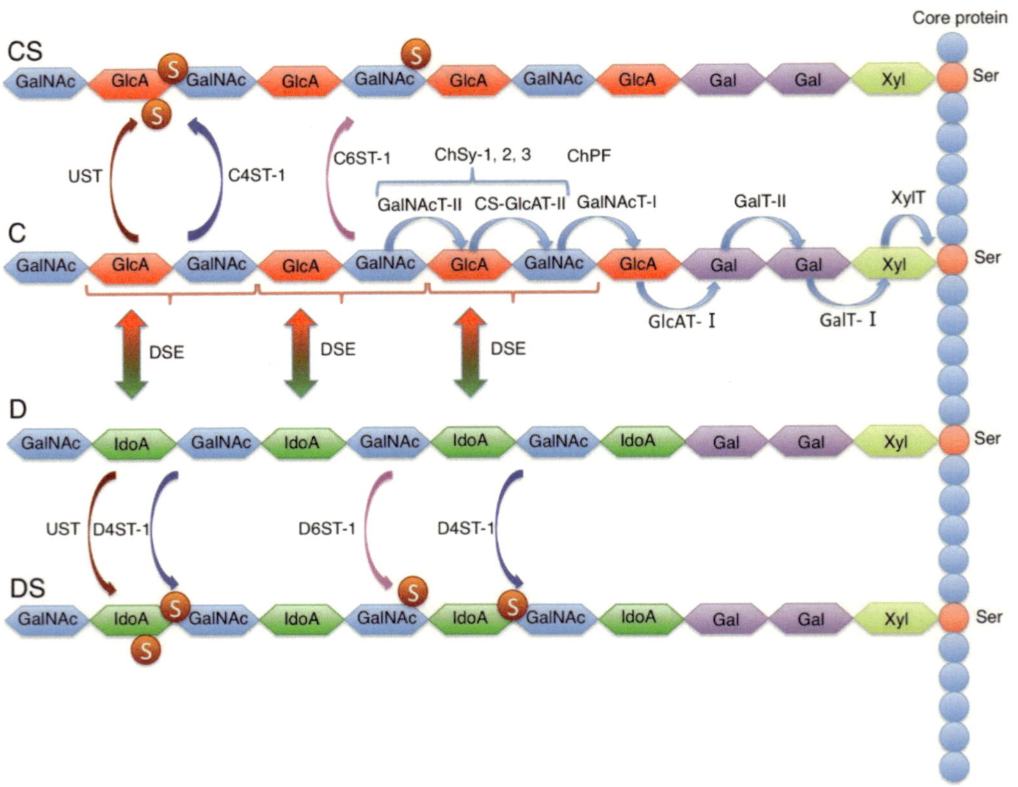

Biosynthesis of chondroitin sulfate (CS) and dermatan sulfate (DS) starts with binding a tetrasaccharide linker region, glucuronic acidβ1-3galactoseβ1-3galactoseβ1-4xyloseβ1-*O*- (GlcA-Gal-Gal-Xyl-), onto serine (Ser) residues of specific core proteins of proteoglycans, by β-xylosyltransferase (XylT), β1,4-galactosyltransferase-I (GalT-I), β1,3-galactosyltransferase-II (GalT-II), and β1,3-glucuronosyltransferase-I (GlcAT-I), respectively. Subsequently, a disaccharide chain of chondroitin (C[N-acetyl-D-galactosamine(GalNAc)-GlcA]$_n$ is synthesized by N-acetyl-D-galactosaminyltransferase-I (GalNAcT-I), N-acetyl-D-galactosaminyltransferase-II (GalNAcT-II), and CS-glucuronyltransferase-II (CS-GlcAT-II) encoded by chondroitin synthase-1, 2, 3 (ChSy-1, 2, 3); and chondroitin polymerizing factor (ChPF). CS chains are matured through sulfation by chondroitin 4-*O*-sulfotransferase-1 (C4ST-1), chondroitin 6-*O*-sulfotransferase-1 (C6ST-1), and uronyl 2-*O*- sulfotransferase (UST). A disaccharide chain of dermatan (D) is synthesized through epimerization of a carboxyl group at C5 from GlcA to L-iduronic acid (IdoA) by dermatan sulfate epimease (DSE). DS chains are matured through sulfation by dermatan 4-*O*-sulfotransferase-1 (D4ST-1), dermatan 6-*O*-sulfotransferase-1 (D6ST-1), and UST. D4ST-1 deficiency, resulting in impaired 4-*O*-sulfation lock, probably allows back epimerization from IdoA to GlcA and finally leads to loss of DS and excess of CS.

Figure 1. Biosynthesis of dermatan sulfate and chondroitin sulfate.

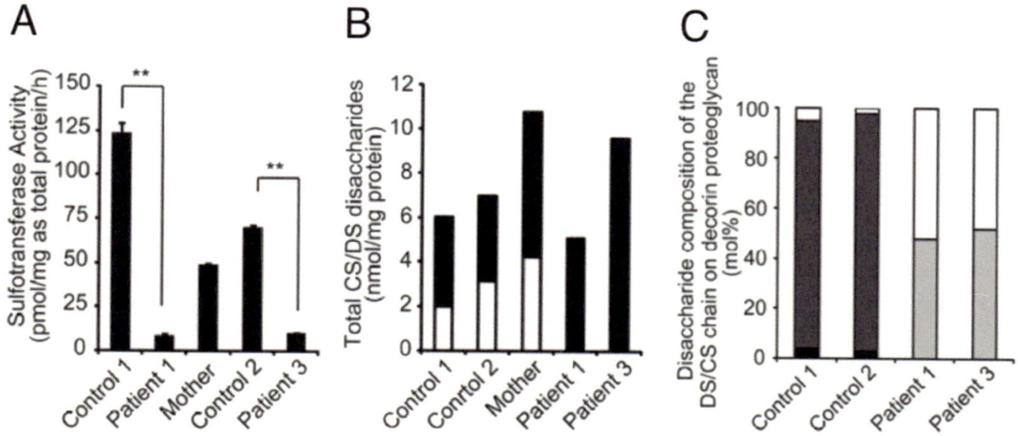

A. Sulfotransferase activity of skin fibroblasts: A patient (a compound heterozygous mutation, P281L/Y293C; patient 1), her heterozygous mother, and her age-matched control (control 1); another patient (a homozygous mutation, P281L; patient 3) and his age-matched control (control 2). B. The total amounts of CS and DS derived from skin fibroblasts. The total disaccharide contents of CS and DS are shown in a black box and a white box, respectively. C. Proportion of the disaccharide units in the CS/DS hybrid chains in decorin secreted by the fibroblasts. A white box and a light gray box indicate GlcUA-GalNAc (4S) and GlcUA-GalNAc (6S), respectively, both composing CS. A dark gray box and a black box indicate IdoUA-GalNAc(4S) and IdoUA-GalNAc (6S), respectively, both composing DS.

Figure 2. Glycobiological studies [6].

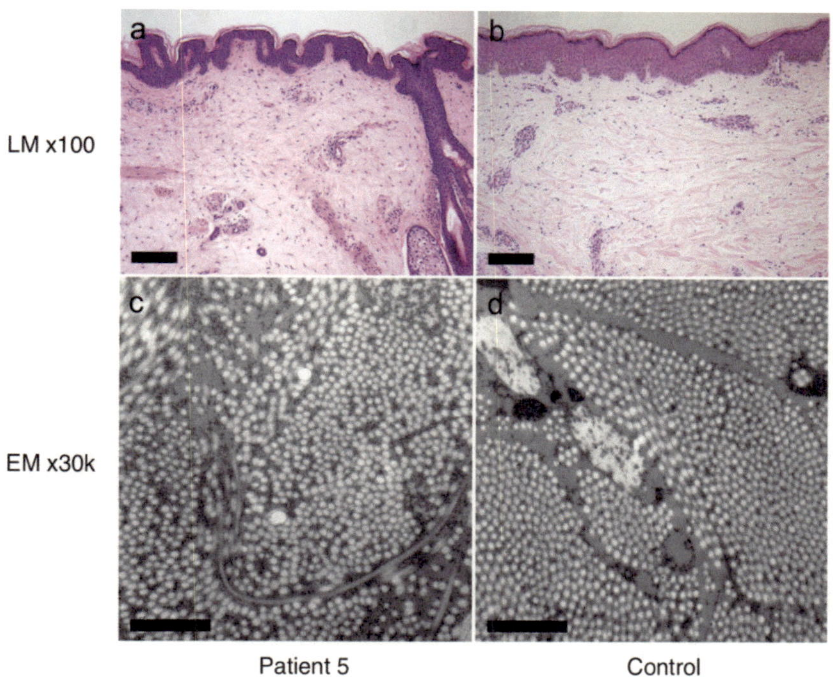

H&E-stained light microscopy (LM) on skin specimens of a patient (a compound heterozygous mutation, P281L/C289S; patient 5) (a) and an age- and sex-matched control (b). Scale bars indicate 500 μm. Electron microscopy (EM) of the patient (c) and the control (d). Scale bars indicate 1 μm.

Figure 3. Pathological studies [6].

In view of these glycobiological and pathological findings, skin fragility in this disorder is suggested to be caused by impaired assembly of collagen fibrils resulting from loss of DS in the GAG chain of decorin [6]. Decorin DS regulates the interfibrillar distance in collagen fibrils and permits the extracellular matrix to resist physical stress, possibly through electrostatic interaction between decorin DS chains and adjacent collagen fibrils (Fig. 4A) [19]. Collagen fibrils are dispersed in patients' skin tissues where the decorin GAG chains are exclusively composed of CS (Fig. 4B), whereas collagen fibrils in controls' skin specimens are tightly assembled through the GAG chains of decorin exclusively composed of DS (Fig. 4A).

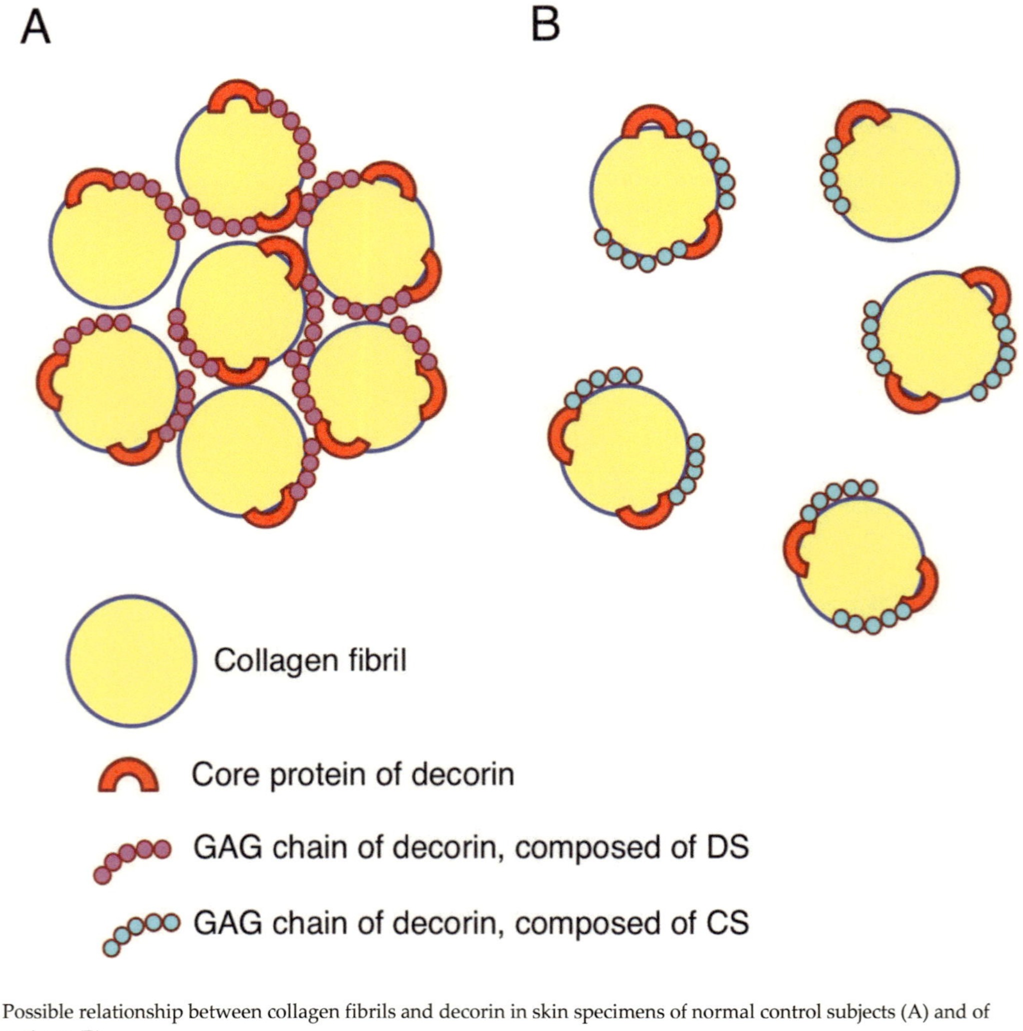

Possible relationship between collagen fibrils and decorin in skin specimens of normal control subjects (A) and of patients (B).

Figure 4. Schema of binding model of decorin to collagen fibrils [20].

4. Delineation of D4ST1-deficient EDS

Independently identified three conditions, ATCS, EDSKT, and MCEDS caused by loss-of-function mutations in CHST14, were supposed to be a single clinically recognizable type of connective tissue disorder [7, 21]. Shimizu et al. [22] presented detailed clinical information of two additional unrelated patients and a comprehensive review of all reported 20 patients, which could definitely unite the three conditions named as "D4ST1-deficient EDS (DD-EDS)". Kosho et al. [23] concluded that categorization of the disorder into a form of "EDS" was appropriate clinically because the disorder satisfied all the hallmarks of EDS including skin hyperextensibility, joint hypermobility, and tissue fragility affecting the skin, ligaments, joints, blood vessels, and internal organs [1] and etiologically because multisystem fragility in the disorder was illustrated to be caused by impaired assembly of collagen fibrils resulting from loss of DS in the decorin GAG chains [6].

To date, 26 patients have been reported to have homozygous or compound heterozygous CHST14 mutations (Table 2) [24, 25, 26]. Clinical characteristics are summarized in Table 3, consisting of progressive multisystem fragility-related manifestations and various malformations [23].

Characteristic craniofacial features including large fontanelle, hypertelorism, short and downslanting palpebral fissures, blue sclerae, short nose with hypoplastic columella, low-set and rotated ears, high palate, long philtrum, thin upper lip vermilion, small mouth, and micro-retrognathia are noted at birth to early childhood (Fig. 5A, B). Slender and asymmetrical facial shapes with protruding jaws are noted from school age (Fig. 5C) [12. 15, 22].

Congenital multiple contractures, most specifically adduction-flexion contractures of thumbs and talipes equinovarus, were cardinal features (Fig. 5D, G, J, K, M). In childhood, peculiar fingers described as "tapering", "slender", and "cylindrical" are also common features (Fig. 5E, F, H, I). Talipes deformities (planus, valgus) (Fig. 5L, N) and spinal deformities (scoliosis, kyphoscoliosis) with tall vertebral bodies and decreased physiological curvature (Fig. 5O, P, Q, R, S, T) occur and progress. Malfanoid habitus, recurrent joint dislocations, and pectus deformities (flat and thin, excavatum, carinatum) are also evident [12. 15, 22].

Cutaneous features include hyperextensibility (Fig. 5U, V) to redundancy (Fig. 5W), bruisability, fragility leading to atrophic scars, acrogeria-like fine palmar creases or wrinkles (Fig. 5F, I), hyperalgesia to pressure, and recurrent subcutaneous infections with fistula formation (Kosho et al., 2005; Kosho et al., 2010; Shimizu et al., 2011).

Recurrent large subcutaneous hematomas are the most serious complication , which sometimes progress acutely and massively to be treated intensively (admission, blood transfusion, surgical drainage) and are supposed to be caused by rupture of subcutaneous arteries or veins (Fig. 5X) [12. 15, 22].

Craniofacial	***Cardiovascular***
Large fontanelle (early choldhood)	Congenital heart defects (ASD)
Hypertelorism	Valve abnormalities (MVP, MR, AR, ARD)
Short and downslanting palpebral fissures	Large subcutaneous hematomas
Blue sclerae	***Gastrointestinal***
Short nose with hypoplastic columella	Constipation
Ear deformities (prominent, posteriorly rotated, low-set)	Diverticula perforation
Palatal abnormalities (high, cleft)	***Respiratory***
Long philtrum and thin upper lip	(Hemo)pneumothorax
Small mouth/micro-retrognathia (infancy)	***Urogenital***
Slender face with protruding jaw (from school age)	Nephrolithiasis/cystolithiasis
Asymmetric face (from school age)	Hydronephrosis
Skeletal	Dilated/atonic bladder
Marfanoid habitus/slender build	Inguinal hernia
Congenital multiple contractures (fingers, wrists, hips, feet)	Cryptorchidism
Recurrent/chronic joint dislocations	Poor breast development
Pectus deformities (flat, excavated)	***Ocular***
Spinal deformities (scoliosis, kyphoscoliosis)	Strabismus
Peculiar fingers (tapering, slender, cylindrical)	Refractive errors (myopia, astigmatism)
Progressive talipes deformilies (valgus, planus, cavum)	Glaucoma/elevated intraocular pressure
Cutaneous	Microcornea/microphthalmia
Hyperextensibility/redundancy	Retinal detachment
Bruisability	***Hearing***
Fragility/atrophic scars	Hearing impairment
Fine/acrogeria-like palmar creases	***Neurological***
Hyperalgesia to pressure	Ventricular enlargement/asymmetry
Recurrent subcutaneous infections/fistula	***Development***
	Hypotonia/gross motor delay.

ASD, atrial septal defect; MVP, mitral valve prolapse; MR, mitral valve regurgitation; AR, aortic valve regurgitation; ARD, aortic rot dilation

Table 3. Clinical manifestations in DD-EDS [23]

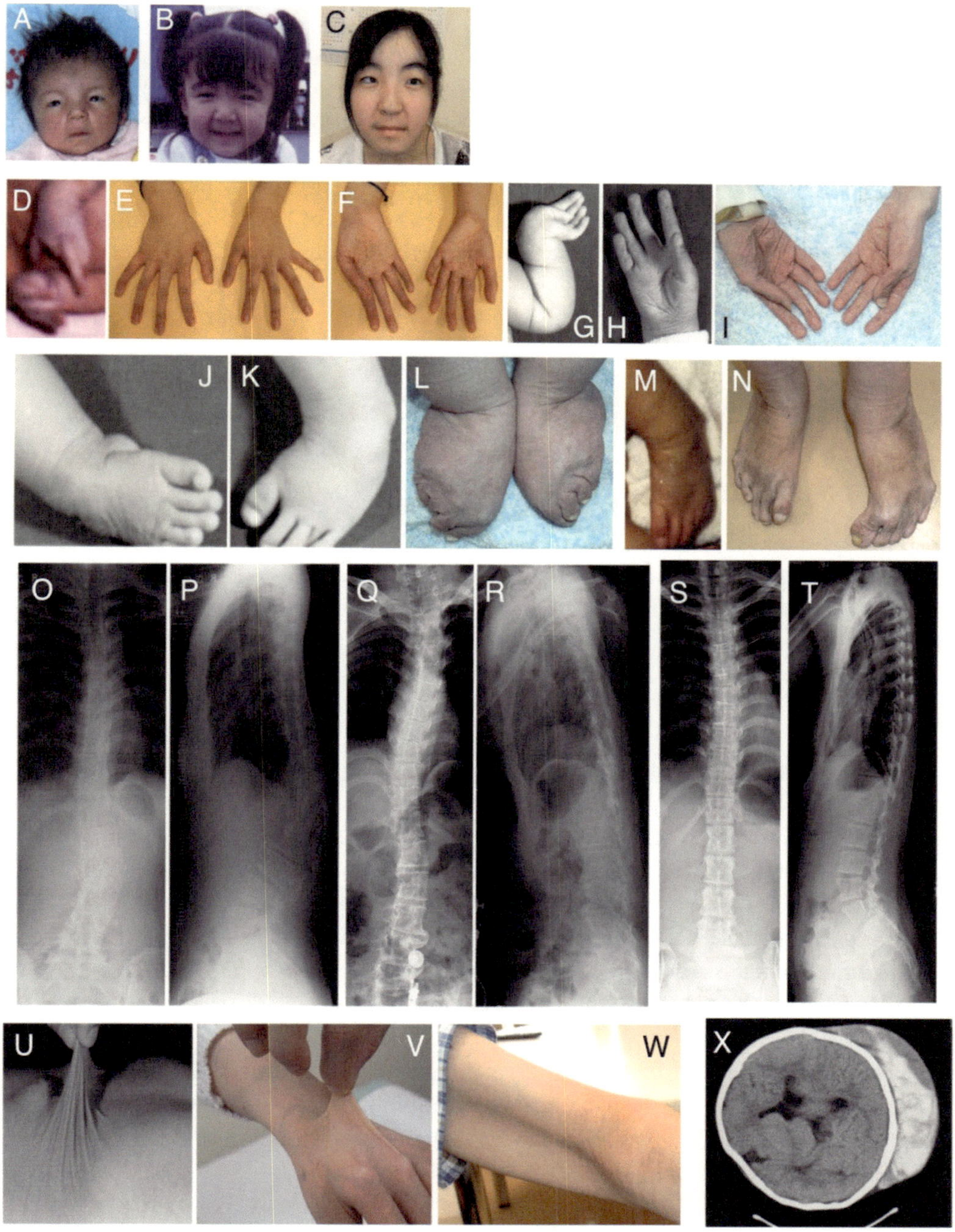

Figure 5. Clinical photographs of patients with DD-EDS [12, 15]. Patient 12 at birth (D), at age 23 days (A), 3 years (B), 6 years (X), and 16 years (C, E, F, O, P). Patient 13 at age 2 months (J, K), 3 months (G), 14 months (U), 5 years (H), and 28 years (I, L, Q, R). Patient 14 in the neonatal period (M) and at age 28 years (N, W). Patient 16 at age 19 years (S, T, V). Patient number is according to Table 2.

5. Conclusion

DD-EDS is a newly recognized and delineated form of EDS, characterized by progressive multisystem fragility-related manifestations (skin hyperextensibilty and fragility, progressive spinal and foot deformities, large subcutaneous hematoma) and various malformations (facial features, congenital eye/heart/gastrointestinal defects, congenital multiple contractures). The cause of multisystem connective tissue fragility is supposed to be impaired assembly of collagen fibrils resulting from loss of DS in the decorin GAG chains. It is the first human disorder affecting biosynthesis of DS, which emphasize a role for DS in human development and extracellular matrix maintenance [27].

Author details

Tomoki Kosho
Department of Medical Genetics, Shinshu University School of Medicine, Asahi, Matsumoto, Japan

Acknowledgement

The author is thankful to all the patients and their families for participating in this study. The authors also express the gratitude to all the collaborators. All the studies were supported by Research on Intractable Diseases from Japanese Ministry of Health, Welfare, and Labor.

6. References

[1] Steinmann B, Royce PM, Superti-Furga A. 2002. The Ehlers–Danlos syndrome. In: Royce PM, Steinmann B, editors. Connective tissue and its heritable disorders. New York: Wiley-Liss, p431–523.

[2] Mao JR, Bristow J. 2001. The Ehlers-Danlos syndrome: on beyond collagens. J Clin Invest 107:1063-1069.

[3] Beighton P, De Paepe A, Steinmann B, Tsipouras P, Wenstrup R. 1998. Ehlers–Danlos syndromes: revised nosology, Villefranche, 1997. Am J Med Genet 77:31–37.

[4] De Paepe A, Malfait F. 2012. The Ehlers-Danlos syndrome, a disorder with many faces. Clin Genet 82:1-11.

[5] Dündar M, Müller T, Zhang Q, Pan J, Steinmann B, Vodopiutz J, Gruber R, Sonoda T, Krabichler B, Utermann G, Baenziger JU, Zhang L, Janecke AR. 2009. Loss of dermatan-4-sulfotransferase 1 function results in adducted thumb-clubfoot syndrome. Am J Hum Genet 85:873–882.

[6] Miyake N, Kosho T, Mizumoto S, Furuichi T, Hatamochi A, Nagashima Y, Arai E, Takahashi K, Kawamura R, Wakui K, Takahashi J, Kato H, Yasui H, Ishida T, Ohashi H, Nishimura G, Shiina M, Saitsu H, Tsurusaki Y, Doi H, Fukushima Y, Ikegawa S, Yamada S, Sugahara K. Matsumoto N. 2010. Loss-of-function mutations of *CHST14* in a new type of Ehles–Danlos syndrome. Hum Mutat 31:966–974.

[7] Malfait F, Syx D, Vlummens P, Symoens S, Nampoothiri S, Hermanns-Lê, Van Lear L, De Paepe A. Musculocontractural Ehlers–Danlos syndrome (former EDS type VIB) and adducted thumb clubfoot syndrome (ATCS) represent a single clinical entity caused by mutations in the dermatan-4-sulfotransferase 1 encoding *CHST14* gene. 2010. Hum Mutat 31:1233–1239.

[8] Dündar M, Demiryilmaz F, Demiryilmaz I, Kumandas S, Erkilic K, Kendirch M, Tuncel M, Ozyazgan I, Tolmie JL. 1997. An autosomal recessive adducted thumb-club foot syndrome observed in Turkish cousins. Clin Genet 51:61–64.

[9] Dündar M, Kurtoglu S, Elmas B, Demiryilmaz F, Candemir Z, Ozkul Y, Durak AC. 2001. A case with adducted thumb and club foot syndrome. Clin Dysmorphol 10:291–293.

[10] Sonoda T, Kouno K. 2000. Two brothers with distal arthrogryposis, peculiar facial appearance, cleft palate, short stature, hydronephrosis, retentio testis, and normal intelligence: a new type of distal arthrogryposis? Am J Med Genet 91:280–285.

[11] Janecke AR, Unsinn K, Kreczy A, Baldissera I, Gassner I, Neu N, Utermann G, Müller T. 2001. Adducted thumb-club foot syndrome in sibs of a consanguineous Austrian family. J Med Genet 38:265–269.

[12] Kosho T, Takahashi J, Ohashi H, Nishimura G, Kato H, Fukushima Y. 2005. Ehlers–Danlos syndrome type VIB with characteristic facies, decreased curvatures of the spinal column, and joint contractures in two unrelated girls. Am J Med Genet Part A 138A:282–287.

[13] Yeowell HN, Steinmann B. 2008. Ehlers-Danlos Syndrome, Kyphoscoliotic Form. n: Pagon RA, Bird TD, Dolan CR, Stephens K, Adam MP, editors. GeneReviews™ [Internet]. Seattle (WA): University of Washington, Seattle; 1993-.2000 Feb 02 [updated 2008 Feb 19].

[14] Yasui H, Adachi Y, Minami T, Ishida T, Kato Y, Imai K. 2003. Combination therapy of DDAVP and conjugated estrogens for a recurrent large subcutaneous hematoma in Ehlers–Danlos syndrome. Am J Hematol 72:71–72.

[15] Kosho T, Miyake N, Hatamochi A, Takahashi J, Kato H, Miyahara T, Igawa Y, Yasui H, Ishida T, Ono K, Kosuda T, Inoue A, Kohyama M, Hattori T, Ohashi H, Nishimura G, Kawamura R, Wakui K, Fukushima Y, Matsumoto N. 2010. A new Ehlers–Danlos syndrome with craniofacial characteristics, multiple congenital contractures, progressive joint and skin laxity, and multisystem fragility-related manifestations. Am J Med Genet Part A 152A:1333–1346.

[16] Evers MR, Xia G, Kang HG, Schachner M, Baeziger JU. 2001. Molecular cloning and characterization of a dermatan-specific *N*-acetylgalactosamine 4-O-sulfotransferase. J Biol Chem 276:36344–36353.

[17] Mikami T, Mizumoto S, Kago N, Kitagawa H, Sugahara K. 2003. Specificities of three distinct human chondroitin/dermatan *N*-acetylgalactosamine 4-O-sulfotransferases demonstrated using partially desulfated dermatan sulfate as an acceptor: implication of differential roles in dermatan sulfate biosynthesis. J Biol Chem 278:36115–36127.

[18] Trowbridge JM, Gallo RL. 2002. Dermatan sulfate: new functions from an old glycosaminoglycan. Glycobiol 12:117R–25R.

[19] Nomura Y. 2006. Structural changes in decorin with skin aging. Connect Tissue Res 47:249–255.

[20] Kosho T. 2011. Discovery and delineation of a new type of Ehlers-Danlos syndrome caused by dermatan 4-*O*-sulfotransferase deficiency. Shinshu Med J 59:305-319.

[21] Janecke AR, Baenziger JU, Müller T, Dündar M. 2011. Letter to the Editors. Loss of dermatan-4-sulfotransferase 1 (D4ST1/*CHST14*) function represents the first dermatan sulfate biosynthesis defect, "Dermatan sulfate-deficient adducted thumb-clubfoot syndrome". Hum Mutat 32:484–485.

[22] Shimizu K, Okamoto N, Miyake N, Taira K, Sato Y, Matsuda K, Akimaru N, Ohashi H, Wakui K, Fukushima Y, Matsumoto N, Kosho T. 2011. Delineation of dermatan 4-O-sulfotransferase 1 deficient Ehlers-Danlos syndrome: observation of two additional patients and comprehensive review of 20 reported patients. Am J Med Genet Part A 155:1949-1958

[23] Kosho T, Miyake N, Mizumoto S, et al. 2011. A response to: loss of dermatan-4-sulfotransferase 1 (D4ST1/CHST14) function represents the first dermatan sulfate biosynthesis defect, "dermatan sulfate-deficient Adducted Thumb-Clubfoot Syndrome". Which name is appropriate, "Adducted Thumb-Clubfoot Syndrome" or "Ehlers-Danlos syndrome"? Hum Mutat 32:1507-1509.

[24] Voermans NC, Kempers M, Lammens M, van Alfen N, Janssen MC, Bönnemann C, van Engelen BG, Hamel BC. 2012. Myopathy in a 20-year-old female patient with D4ST-1 deficient Ehlers-Danlos syndrome due to a homozygous CHST14 mutation. Am J Med Genet A 158A:850-855.

[25] Mendoza-Londono R, Chitayat D, Kahr WH, Hinek A, Blaser S, Dupuis L, Goh E, Badilla-Porras R, Howard A, Mittaz L, Superti-Furga A, Unger S, Nishimura G, Bonafe L. 2012. Extracellular matrix and platelet function in patients with musculocontractural Ehlers-Danlos syndrome caused by mutations in the *CHST14* gene. Am J Med Genet A 158A:1344-1354.

[26] Winters KA, Jiang Z, Xu W, Li S, Ammous Z, Jayakar P, Wierenga KJ. 2012. Re-assigned diagnosis of D4ST1-deficient Ehlers-Danlos syndrome (adducted thumb-clubfoot syndrome) after initial diagnosis of Marden-Walker syndrome. Am J Med Genet A 158A:2935-2940.

[27] Zhang L, Müller T, Baenziger JU, Janecke AR. 2010. Congenital disorders of glycosylation with emphasis on loss of dermatan-4-sulfotransferase? 93:289–307.

Chapter 7

Eryhtropoietic Protoporphyria

Akira Kawada, Shigeru Kawara and Hajime Nakano

Additional information is available at the end of the chapter

http://dx.doi.org/10.5772/54132

1. Introduction

The porphyrias are metabolism diseases caused by the deficiency of a specific enzyme in the heme biosynthetic pathway. Porphyrias have been classified into bone marrow and liver types on the basis of the predominant site of porphyrin production site. Recent classification of porphyrias shows acute porphyria and cutaneous porphyria according to the condition of signs (Table 1). Eryhtropoietic protoporphyria (EPP; OMIM 177000) is an autosomal dominant disease of porphyrin metabolism caused by decreased activity of the ferrochelatase (FECH; E.C. 4.99.1.1) that is the terminal enzyme in the heme biosynthetic pathway (Fig. 1). This type of porphyria was first described in 1953 by Kosenow and Treibs and this description was completed in 1961 by Magnus et al.[1] Decrease in FECH activity causes excess protoporphyrin induction, leading to photosensitivity of the skin and liver dysfunction. Photosensitivity starting from childhood makes quality of life low and liver dysfunction may lead to hepatic failure and death. In this session, we describe (1) clinical features of EPP, (2) genetic characteristics of EPP, and (3) mice models of EPP.

2. The clinical features of EPP

2.1. Skin

Suspicion of EPP should be raised by the history of screaming or skin pain in a child on going outdoors.[2] However, it is very difficult to suspect EPP if clinical manifestation are minimum. The characteristics of photosensitivity in EPP are first a burning, stinging sensation appearing immediately at sun exposure followed by erythema, edema and purpura.[1] We reported a 1-year-old male infant with EPP who showed only erythema after sun exposure (Fig. 2).[3] Infant patients are unable to complain the abnormal sensations and pain. Cutaneous signs are characterized with erythema, swelling, papules, vesicles, small blood blisters, crusts, and scars. Scar, the most distinct skin lesion, is small, polygonal or linear, depressed or slightly elevated (Figs. 3 and 4). With the progression of the disease and

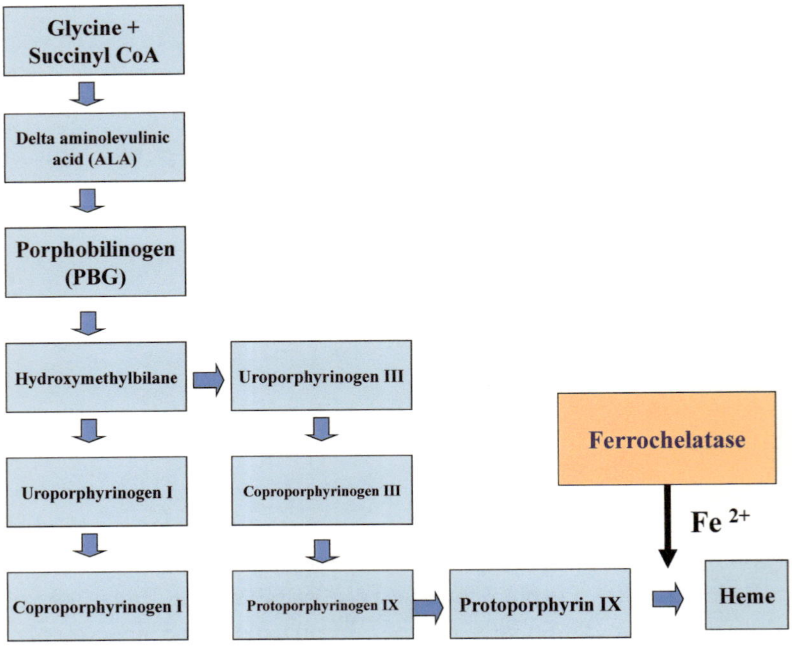

Figure 1. Heme biosynthetic pathway.

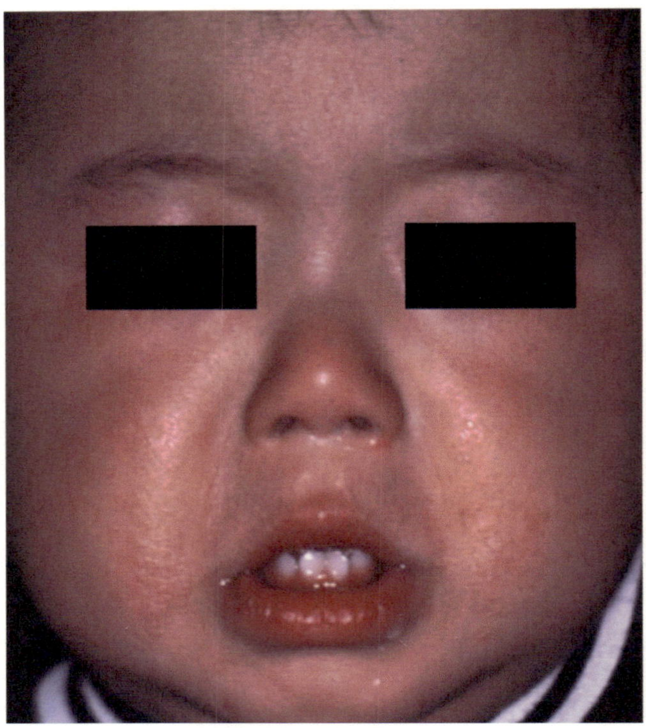

Figure 2. Clinical picture of a 1-year-old male baby with erythopoietic protoporphyria. Redness and swelling were seen on the face.

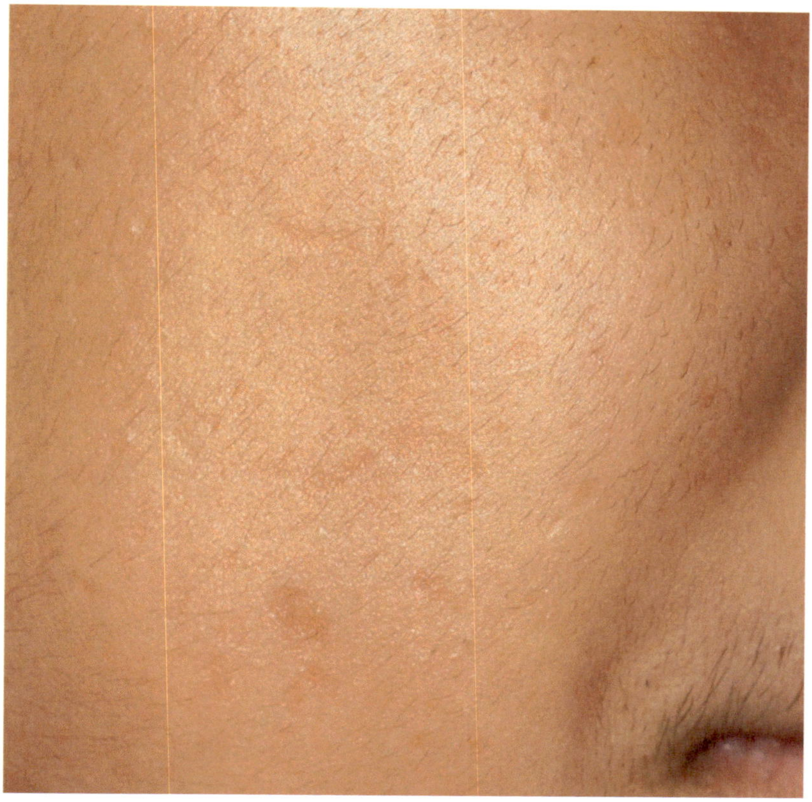

Figure 3. Clinical picture of a 14-year-old boy with erythopoietic protoporphyria. Depressed scars were seen on the face.

if sun exposure is not avoided, chronic lesions develop progressively with skin thickening (waxy lichenification on the dorsa of the hands) and scarring (pseudorhagades formation in the lips).[1]

Minder performed a systematic review of treatment options for dermal photosensitivity in EPP.[4] Sixteen of 25 relevant studies dealed with β-carotene. However, the results from β-carotene were strongly contradictory and efficacy was inversely correlated with study quality.[4] Afamelanotide, an a-melanocyte-stimulating hormone analogue, was reported to be effective for EPP.[5] Afamelanotide, making melanin density of the skin increase, was effective for photosensitivity from artificial light and sunlight in 5 EPP patients.[5] Moreover, Petersen reported that oral treatment with a high daily dosage of zinc sulphate during the spring and summer reduced light sensitivity and pain in 71% of 14 EPP patients.[6] They speculated that zinc treatment in EPP patients may have provided antioxidant protection of cellular membranes against the deleterious photodynamic effects of protoporphyrin IX (PPIX) accumulation.[6] Photoprotection against visible light that absorbs PPIX is still a mainstream in the care of EPP patients, although these novel approaches were reported. However, some reports raised awareness about vitamin D deficiency due to sun avoidance in EPP. Spelt reported that 46% of 48 Dutch EPP patients showed decreased level of serum

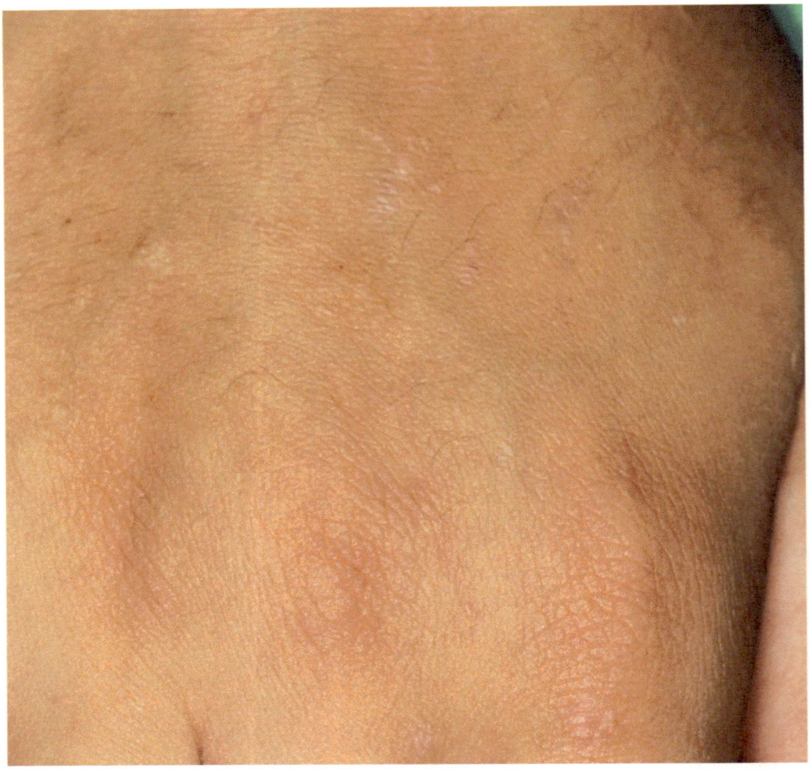

Figure 4. Clinical picture of a 14-year-old boy with erythopoietic protoporphyria. Whitish swelling scars were seen on the back of the hand.

25-hydroxyvitamin D.[7] Vitamin D deficiency was high in male patients and correlated with the severity of EPP.[7] Holme also reported that 17% was deficient and 63% was insufficient in serum 25-hydroxyvitamin D levels of 201 United Kingdom (UK) patients with EPP.[8] Then, we should care for vitamin D deficiency in EPP patients performing strict photoprotection.

2.2. Liver

Mild abnormalities of liver function may be detected in about 10% of patients of EPP and liver failure affects about 5-20%.[2, 9] Excess PP with any origin is excreted by the liver into bile and enters an enterohepatic circulation.[10] Excess PP becomes insoluble in bile and exerts cholestatic effects, structural changes from mild inflammation to fibrosis and cirrhosis.[10] Liver diseases include cholelithiasis, gallstones, biochemical abnormalities (aspartate amino transferase (AST), alanine amino transferase (ALT), gamma-glutamyl transpeptidase (gamma-GTP), alkaline phosphatase (ALP)), cirrhosis, and terminal liver failure. PP deposition in hepatocytes is invariable, whereas histological evidence of damage is less common; electron microscopy shows ultrastructural damage in most patients with EPP.[10]

Liver transplantation for liver failure in EPP patients started in 1980. Dowman investigated 5 UK cases receiving liver transplant for EPP-related liver diseases.[11] Two patients died at 44 and 95 months from causes unrelated to liver disease, while 3 patients were alive at 22.4 years, 61 months and 55 months after liver plant.[11] In spite of a good long-term survival, a high rate of postoperative biliary stricturing requiring multiple biliary interventions was seen.[11] Wahlin also investigated that 35 liver transplants for protoporphyric liver disease in 31 European patients between 1983 and 2008.[12] The overall rate of disease recurrence in the graft was high (69%), although they showed good survival rates, 77% at 1 year and 66% at 5 and 10 years.[12]

As liver transplant does not correct the constitutional deficiency of FECH, there is a risk of recurrence of liver disease even after liver transplant due to continuing overproduction of protoporphyrin.[9] Then, bone marrow transplantation may be considered in liver allograft recipients in the future.

2.3. Biochemistry and blood test

Increase of PP in the blood and stool is the most specific in EPP. However, urinary porphyris (uroporphyrin, coproporphyrin, porphobirinoge, δ-aminolevulic acid) remain as normal levels. Many patients with EPP have an apparent mild anemia with a microcytic hypochromic blood film.[2] However, administration of iron is not recommended since iron sometimes exacerbate the porphyria.

3. Genetic characteristics of EPP

EPP is a disease caused by decreased activity of the ferrochelatase (FECH; E.C. 4.99.1.1) that is the final enzyme in the heme biosynthetic pathway. The *FECH* gene contains 11 exons and spans about 45 kb of genomic DNA on chromosome 18q21.3, and its cDNA sequence encodes for 423 amino acids (GenBank no. D00726). The mode of inheritance is primarily autosomal dominant, and the clinical penetrance is low. In the dominant type of EPP, different degrees of enzyme deficiency are seen between patients and asymptomatic gene carriers, *i.e.*, symptomatic patients usually have less than 50% of the normal activity, whereas the asymptomatic ones show approximately 50% of the normal activity.[13]

Gouya reported that (1) coinheritance of a *FECH* gene defect and a wild-type low-expressed allele is generally involved in the clinical expression of EPP; (2) the low-expressed allelic variant was associated with a partial 5′ haplotype [-251G IVS1-23T IVS2μsatA9] that may be ancestral and was present in an estimated 10% of a control group of Caucasian origin; and (3) haplotyping allows the absolute risk of developing the disease to be predicted for those inheriting *FECH* EPP mutations.[13] Mutations of *FECH* gene in EPP are highly heterogenous and specific for each family members. Minder studied the association between "null allele" mutation and liver complication in 1112 EPP patients.[14] All 18 EPP patients who had severe liver complication showed a "null allele" mutation, whereas 20 patients with a missense mutation did not have liver complication till the time of study.[14] This study indicates that a significant genotype-phenotype correlation between "null allele" mutation and liver disorder in EPP.

Genetic variants in the *FECH* gene include more than 175 mutations and 538 single-nucleotide polymorphisms (SNPs).[15] The functionality of these SNPs may reduce the level of transcription of the *FECH* gene contributing to the triggering of EPP.[15] A common low expression allele, IVS3-48T>C, is seen in 10% of European Caucasians. Most EPP patients (~90%) have a *FECH* loss-of-function mutation *in cis* and the common low expression allele *in trans*, resulting in 15-25% of normal FECH activity.[16] As described above, mutations of *FECH* gene in EPP are highly family-specific. There have been many variations of *FECH* gene mutations reported in various countries.

Nakano firstly identified two novel mutations in two Japanese families using direct sequence analysis of the entire coding region of the FECH gene.[17] The proband in the first family was heterozygous for a 3-bp deletion from nucleotide positions 853 to 855 in exon 8, designated delCAA^{853}.[17] Pedigree analysis of the other family members showed that the mother and two sisters, all asymptomatic, were heterozygous for this mutation.[17] Restriction fragment polymorphism analysis indicated that the proband was homozygous for the IVS3-48C polymorphism, while other family members, asymptomatic carriers, had a wild-type T at position IVS3-48 in *trans* to the mutated allele.[17] They concluded that the IVS3-48C polymorphism in one allele and a deleterious mutation (delCAA^{853}) in the other allele caused a phenotype of EPP. In the second family, all three members having symptoms of EPP showed the C^{683}→T mutation in combination with the trans IVS3-48C polymorphism.[17] These results from the analysis of two Japanese families indicated that the intronic IVS3-48C polymorphism in the non-mutated allele is a distinct determinant of the EPP phenotype. Their further investigation of the frequency of IVS-48C polymorphism in 104 Japanese controls revealed that the genotypic frequency of IVS3-48C/C was 0.192, that was over 10 times those of European countries (0-0.017).[17] These differences may affect the prevalence and penetrance of EPP in Japan.

In UK, Whatley identified large deletions of the *FECH* gene in 19 (58%) of 33 unrelated UK patients with EPP using gene dosage analysis by quantitative PCR; (1) six deletions (c.1-7887-IVS1+ 2425insTTCA; c.1-9629-IVS1+ 2437; IVS2-1987-IVS4+352del; c.768-IVS7+ 244del; IVS7+2784-IVS9+108del; IVS6+2350-TGA+95del), (2) five breakpoints in intronic repeat sequences (AluSc, AluSq, AluSx, L1MC4), and (3) large insertion-deletion (Del Ex3-4).[18] Berroeta reported a UK case with late onset of EPP and identified a mutation (1001C→T; P334L).[19]

In Canada, Pierro identified a 10,376 bp deletion (c.1-7887_67+2422del) including a portion of the upstream intergenic region, the promoter, the exon 1 and a portion of intron 1 in a Canadian EPP patient of Italian origin.[20] Li also reported that a Canadian EPP patient had a novel large deletion [c.1-9628_67+2871del12566 bp] and three polymorphisms [c.1-251A>G, c.68-23C>T and c.315-48T>C] in trans to the deletion in *FECH* gene.[21]

In China, Zhou identified a novel IVS1+1G→C mutation of the FECH gene in a Chinese EPP family.[22] Fong identified a recurrent splice site mutation, c.67+1G>C, and a novel nonsense mutation, p.Y191X, in 2 unrelated Chinese families.[23] Their investigation revealed that the allele frequency of IVS3-48C in Hong Kong population (28%) was lower than that of

Japanese population but higher than that of European populations.[23] Ma identified a novel splicing *FECH* mutation, IVS3+1G→A, and IVS3-48C polymorphism in a Chinese EPP family.[24]

In Argentina, Parera detected three novel and two previously described mutations in five Argentinean EPP families; (1) a deletion (451delT) producing a stop codon located 18 codons downstream from the mutation, (2) IVS1-2A>G leading to exon 2 skipping, (3) IVS4-2A>G, which causes the loss of the first 48 bp of exon 5, (4) C343T, and (5) 400delA.[25] Colombo's study of 19 Argentina EPP patients identified three novel (p.S222N; p.R298X and p.R367X) and seven already known (g.12490_18067del; p.R115X; p.I186T; c.580_584delTACAG; c.598+1G>T; p.Y209X and p.W310X) and indicated the possibility of c.315-48C variant in *trans* to the mutated allele as a sufficient trigger of EPP.[15]

In Spain, Herrero reported that three novel mutations (IVS4+1delG, 347-351delC, and 130_147dupl 18) and IVS3-48C low-expression allele in ten of 11 EPP patients.[26] They also estimated the frequency of the IVS3-48C allele among 180 nonporphyric Spanish individuals as 5.2%.[26] In South Africa, Parker identified ten sequence variations; IVS3-48T / C polymorphism, five further polymorphisms, a 5-bp deletion in exon 7 (757_761delAGAAG), two previously described splice-site mutations (IVS3+2T>G and IVS7+1G>A), and a novel 7-bp deletion in exon 4 (356_362delTTCAAGA).[27] In Portugal, Morais identified heterozygosity for a novel mutation (c.1052delA) in *FECH* gene of two children, and heterozygosity for the hypomorphic allele IVS3-48T>C in two children and asymptomatic mother.[28]

Recently, an association of EPP and palmar keratoderma has been reported. Méndez detected a homozygous inheritance of a novel missense mutation Q285R, a homozygous A-to-G transition, c.854A>G, in the *FECH* gene in a Caucasian family of EPP associated with palmar keratoderma.[29] Minder also reported a case of an association of EPP and palmar keratoderma who had a novel homoallelic missense mutation (p.Ser318Tyr) in the *FECH* gene.[30] Their Palestinial (Jordanian) parents were heterozygous for the S318Y mutation.[30]

4. Mice models of EPP

Mice models of EPP are useful to investigate the effects of FECH on iron metabolism in EPP. Lyoumi investigated hematologic and iron status in FECH-deficient Fechm1Pas mutant mice.[31] Their mice had microcytic hypochromic anemia without ringed sideroblasts, little or no hemolysis, and no erythroid hyperplasia, whereas the mice showed no tissue iron deficiency but did a redistribution of iron stores from peripheral tissues to the spleen, with a 2- to 3-fold increase in transferrin expression of mRNA and protein levels.[31] Using Fechm1Pas mutant mice with the BALB/c and C57BL/6 backgrounds, Lyoumi demonstrated that BALB/c backgrounded Fechm1Pas mice had more severe cholestasis, fibrosis with portoportal bridging, bile acid regurgitation, sclerosing cholangitis, and hepatolithiasis as compared with the mice with C57BL/6 background.[32]

5. Conclusion

EPP is an autosomal dominant disease of porphyrin metabolism that is characterized with photosensitivity and liver disease. We have reviewed recent advances of clinical features of EPP, genetic characteristics of EPP, and mice models of EPP. Further studies of genetic analysis and FECH-deficient mice will provide us the new strategy for the treatment of EPP.

Author details

Akira Kawada
Department of Dermatology, Kinki University Faculty of Medicine, Osaka-Sayama, Osaka, Japan

Shigeru Kawara
Department of Dermatology, Kanazawa Red Cross Hospital, Kanazawa, Japan

Hajime Nakano
Department of Dermatology, Hirosaki University School of Medicine, Hirosaki, Aomori, Japan

6. References

[1] Lecha M. Eryhtropoietic protoporphyria. Photodermatol Photomed Photoimmunol 2003; 19: 142-6.
[2] Murphy GM. Diagnosis and management of the erythropoietic protoporphyris. Dermatol Ther 2003; 16: 57-64.
[3] Kawada A, Gomi H, Shiraishi H, Hatanaka K, Matsuo I, Inafuku K, Takamori K, Tezuka T. An infantile case of erythropoietic protoporphyria with a decreased mRNA level of ferrocheratase. Hifu 2001; 43: 111-5.
[4] Minder EI, Schneider-Yin X, Steurer J, Bachmann LM. A systematic review of treatment options for dermal photosensitivity in erythropoietic protoporphyria. Cell Mol Biol 2009; 55: 84-97.
[5] Harms J, Lautenschlager S, Minder CE, Minder EI. An α-melanocyte–stimulating hormone analogue in erythropoietic protoporphyria. N Eng J Med 2009; 360: 306-7.
[6] Petersen AB, Philipsen PA, Wulf HC. Zinc sulphate: a new concept of treatment of erythropoietic protoporphyria. Br J Dermatol 2012; 166: 1129-31.
[7] Spelt JMC, Rooij FWM, Wilson JHP, Zandbergen AAM. Vitamin D deficiency in patients with erythropoietic protoporphyria. J Inherit Metab Dis 2009 doi: 10.1007/s10545-008-1037-0.
[8] Holme SA, Anstey AV, Badminton MN, Elder GH. Serum 25-hydroxyvitamin D in erythropoietic protoporphyria. Br J Dermatol 2008; 159: 211-3.
[9] Casanova-González MJ, Trapero-Marugán M, Jones EA, Moreno-Otero R. Liver disease and erythropoietic protoporphyria: a concise review. World J Gastroenterol. 2010; 16: 4526-31.
[10] Anstey AV, Hift RJ. Liver disease in erythropoietic protoporphyria: insights and implications for management. Gut 2007; 56: 1009-18.

[11] Dowman JK, Gunson BK, Mirza DF, Badminton MN, Newsome PN. UK experience of liver transplantation for erythropoietic protoporphyria. J Inherit Metab Dis 2011; 34: 539-45.

[12] Wahlin S, Stal P, Adam R, Karam V, Porte R, Seehofer D, Gunson BK, Hillingsø J, Klempnauer JL, Schmidt J, Alexander G, O'Grady J, Clavien PA, Salizzoni M, Paul A, Rolles K, Ericzon BG, Harper P. Liver transplantation for erythropoietic protoporphyria in Europe. Liver Transpl 2011; 17: 1021-6.

[13] Gouya L, Puy H, Lamoril J, Silva VD, Grandchamp B, Nordmann Y, Deybach J-C. Inheritance in erythropoietic protoporphyria: a common wild-type ferrochelatase allelic variant with low expression accounts for clinical manifestation. Blood 1999; 93: 2105-10.

[14] Minder EI, Gouya L, Schneider-Yin X, Deybach JC. A genotype-phenotype correlation between null-allele mutations in the ferrochelatase gene and liver complication in patients with erythropoietic protoporphyria. Cell Mol Biol 2002; 48: 91-6.

[15] Colombo FP, Rossetti MV, Méndez M, Martínez JE, Enríquez de Salamanca R, Batlle AMC, Parera VE. Functional associations of genetic variants involved in the clinical manifestation of erythropoietic protoporphyria in the argentinean population. J Eur Acad Dermatol Venereol 2012 doi: 10.1111/j.1468-3083.2012.04566.x.

[16] Balwani M, Desnick RJ. The porphyrias: advances in diagnosis and treatment. Blood 2012 doi:10.1182/blood-2012-05-423186

[17] Nakano H, Nakano A, Toyomaki Y, Ohashi S, Harada K, Moritsugu R, Takeda H, Kawada A, Mitsuhashi Y, Hanada K. Novel Ferrochelatase Mutations in Japanese Patients with erythropoietic protoporphyria: high frequency of the splice site modulator IVS3-48C polymorphism in the Japanese population. J Invest Dermatol 2006; 126: 2717-9.

[18] Whatley SD, Mason NG, Holme SA, Anstey AV, Elder GH, Badminton MN. Gene dosage analysis identifies large deletions of the *FECH* gene in 10% of families with erythropoietic protoporphyria. J Invest Dermatol 2007; 127: 2790-4.

[19] Berroeta L, Man I, Goudie DR, Whatley SD, Elder GH, Ibbotson SH. Late presentation of erythropoietic protoporphyria: case report and genetic analysis of family members. Br J Dermatol 2007; 157: 1030-1.

[20] Di Pierro E, Brancaleoni V, Besana V, Ausenda S, Drury S, Cappellini MD. A 10376 bp deletion of FECH gene responsible for erythropoietic protoporphyria. Blood Cells Mol Dis 2008; 40: 233-6.

[21] Li C, Di Pierro E, Brancaleoni V, Cappellini MD, Steensma DP. A novel large deletion and three polymorphism in the FECH gene associated with erythropoietic protoporphyria. Clin Chem lab Med 2009; 47: 44-6.

[22] Zhou SN, Xiao SX, Peng ZH, Li BX, Li XL, Li Y, Luo SJ. A novel mutation of the FECH gene in a Chinese family with erythropoietic protoporphyria. J Dermatol Sci 2007; 48: 145-7.

[23] Lau KC, Lam CW. DNA-based diagnosis of erythropoietic protoporphyria in two families and the frequency of a low-expression *FECH* allele in a Chinese population. Clin Chim Acta 2009; 400: 132-4.

[24] Ma J, Xiao S, An J, Wang X, Xu Q, Dong Y, Feng Y, Wang J. A novel splicing mutation and haplotype analysis of the *FECH* gene in a Chinese family with erythropoietic protoporphyria. J Eur Acad Dermatol Venereol 2010; 24: 726-9.

[25] Parera VE, Koole RH, Minderman G, Edixhoven A, Rossetti MV, Batlle A, De Rooij FWM. Novel null-allele mutations and genotype-phenotype correlation in Argentinean patients with erythropoietic protoporphyria. Mol Med 2009; 15: 425-31.

[26] Herrero C, To-Figueras J, Badenas C, Méndez M, Serrano P, Enríquez-Salamanca R, Lecha M. Clinical, biochemical, and genetic study of 11 patients with erythropoietic protoporphyria including one with homozygous disease. Arch Dermatol 2007; 143: 1125-9.

[27] Parker M, Corrigall AV, Hift RJ, Meissner PN. Molecular characterization of erythropoietic protoporphyria in South Africa. Br J Dermatol 2008; 159: 182-91.

[28] Morais P, Mota A, Baudrier T, Trigo F, Oliveira JP, Cerqueira R, Palmeiro A, Tavares P, Azevedo F. Erythropoietic protoporphyria: a family study and report of a novel mutation in the FECH gene. Eur J Dermatol 2011; 21: 479-83.

[29] Méndez M, Poblete-Gutiérrez P, Morán-Jiménez MJ, Rodriguez ME, Garrido-Astray MC, Fontanellas A, Frank J, de Salamanca RE. A homozygous mutation in the ferrochelatase gene underlies erythropoietic protoporphyria associated with palmar keratoderma. Br J Dermatol 2009; 160: 1330-4.

[30] Minder EI, Schneider-Yin X, Mamet R, Horev L, Neuenschwander S, Baumer A, Austerlitz F, Puy H, Schoenfeld N. A homoallelic FECH mutation in a patient with both erythropoietic protoporphyria and palmar keratoderma. J Eur Acad Dermatol Venereol 2010; 24: 1349-53.

[31] Lyoumi S, Abitbol M, Andrieu V, Henin D, Robert E, Schmitt C, Gouya L, de Verneuil H, Deybach JC, Montagutelli X, Beaumont C, Puy H. Increased plasma transferrin, altered body iron distribution, and microcytic hypochromic anemia in ferrochelatase-deficient mice. Blood 2007; 109: 811-8.

[32] Lyoumi S, Abitbol M, Rainteau D, Karim Z, Bernex F, Oustric V, Millot S, Letteron P, Heming N, Guillmot L, Montagutelli X, Berdeaux G, Gouya L, Poupon R, Deybach JC, Beaumont C, Puy H. Protoporphyrin retention in hepatocytes and Kupffer cells prevents sclerosing cholangitis in erythropoietic protoporphyria mouse model. Gastroenterology 2011; 141: 1509–19.

Chapter 8

Hermansky-Pudlak Syndrome

Naoki Oiso and Akira Kawada

Additional information is available at the end of the chapter

http://dx.doi.org/10.5772/53573

1. Introduction

Oculocutaneous albinism is classified into non-syndromic oculocutaneous albinism (OCA) and syndromic OCA including Hermansky-Pudlak syndrome (HPS), Chediak-Higashi syndrome (CHS) and Griscelli syndrome (GS). Both non-syndromic and syndromic OCAs are autosomal recessive disorders. Human HPS is genetically divided into nine forms, HPS type 1 (HPS-1) to HPS-9. Human HPS can be sub-classified into four subgroups which are associated with protein complexes encoded by the causative genes. In this session, we summarize (1) the clinical features of HPS, (2) the mice and rat models of HPS, and (3) the molecular functions.

2. The clinical features of HPS

In 1959, Hermansky and Pudklak described two cases of OCA associated with hemorrhagic diathesis.[1] Currently, the condition is known as HPS. HPS is a rare heterogeneous autosomal recessive syndrome which is typically characterized by OCA, bleeding diathesis, and lysosomal ceroid storage resulting from defects of multiple cytoplasmic organelles: melanosomes, platelet dense core granules, and lysosomes.[2] The storage of ceroid-like material in lysosomes induces restrictive lung disease, ulcerative colitis, kidney failure, and cardiomyopathy.

Accumulation of mice models, identification of causative genes and functional analysis indicated that HPS could be sub-classified into four groups according to four protein complexes, biogenesis of lysosome-related organelles complex-3 (BLOC-3) (HPS-1 and HPS-4), adaptor protein-3 (AP-3) (HPS-2), BLOC-2 (HPS-3, HPS-5 and HPS-6) and BLOC-1(HPS-7, HPS-8 and HPS-9).[3-5] Currently, more than 16 mice strains and more than 2 rat strains are known as models of human HPS (**Table 1**). HPS-1 is caused by mutation in *HPS1*,[6] HPS-2 is caused by mutation in *AP3B1*,[7] HPS-3 is caused by mutation in *HPS3*,[8] HPS-4 is caused by mutation in *HPS4*,[9] HPS-5 is caused by mutation in *HPS5*,[10] HPS-6 is caused by mutation in

HPS6,[10] HPS-7 is caused by mutation in *DTNBP1*,[11] HPS-8 is caused by mutation in *BLOC1S3*,[12] and HPS-9 is caused by mutation in *PLDN*.[13] Functional analyses identify that most of all HPS proteins construct complexes, BLOC-1, BLOC-2, BLOC-3, AP3, class C vacuolar protein sorting (VPS), and Rab geranylgeranyl transferase (RABGGT).

Mouse models	**Human type**	**Genes**	**Protein complexes**
pale ear	HPS-1	*HPS1*	BLOC-3
pearl	HPS-2	*AP3B1*	AP3
cocoa	HPS-3	*HPS3*	BLOC-2
light ear	HPS-4	*HPS4*	BLOC-3
ruby-eye-2	HPS-5	*HPS5*	BLOC-2
ruby-eye	HPS-6	*HPS6*	BLOC-2
sandy	HPS-7	*DTNBP1*	BLOC-1
reduced pigmentation	HPS-8	*BLOC1S3*	BLOC-1
pallid	HPS-9	*PLDN*	BLOC-1
buff	?	*VPS33A*	class C VPS
cappuccino	?	*CNO*	BLOC-1
gunmetal	?	*RABGGTA*	RABGGT
misty	?	*DOCK7*	
mocha	?	*AP3D1*	AP3
muted	?	*MUTED*	BLOC-1
subtle gray	?	*SLC7A11*	
Rat models			
Fawn-Hooded rat	?	*RAB38*	
Tester-Moriyama rat	?	*RAB38*	

Table 1. Animal models, human types, causative genes and their protein complexes in HPS.

HPS-1 and HPS-4, the group of BLOC-3, are the most dominant and typical subtypes. The founder effect in HPS-1 is present in the region of northwest Puerto Rico.[8] HPS-1 and HPS-4 are characterized by OCA by deficiency of melanosomes, bleeding by loss of platelet dense core granules, and systemic organ involvement (restrictive lung disease, granulomatous colitis, kidney failure, and cardiomyopathy) by the storage of lysosomal ceroid-like substances due to impaired lysosomes. The clinical features of OCA and bleeding diathesis are present in infancy. Bleeding tendency is important to diagnose.

HPS-2, the group of AP3, is the most severe and rare subtype, with 15 cases reported in the literature.[14] Clinical manifestations include OCA, a platelet storage pool defect, interstitial lung disease, and recurrent bacterial and viral infections due to immunodeficiency.[14] Patients with HPS-2 exhibit neutropenia that is responsive to granulocyte colony-stimulation factor, deficiency of natural killer and natural killer T-cells, T-lymphocyte dysfunction, and in one case hemophagocytic lymphohistiocytosis.[14]

HPS-3, HPS-5, and HPS-6, the group of BLOC-2, are the milder and relatively rare subtypes. The founder effect in HPS-3 is present in the area of central Puerto Rico.[8] HPS-3, HPS-5 and HPS-6 are relatively milder forms of the disease in that both OCA and bleeding diathesis are mild and pulmonary fibrosis and granulomatous colitis generally does not develop.[10, 15-17]

HPS-7, HPS-8, and HPS-9, the group of BLOC-1, are extremely rare subtypes. HPS-7 is only found in a 48-year-old Portuguese woman with OCA, a bleeding tendency, mild shortness of breath on exertion and reduced lung compliance but otherwise normal pulmonary function.[11] HPS-8 is found in a Pakistani family[12] and an Iranian patient.[18] HPS-8 is characterized by typical OCA and a bleeding diathesis. Pulmonary fibrosis, granulomatous colitis, or neutropenia are not detected in the cases. [12, 18] HPS-9 is only found in a 9-month-old male of Indian ancestry.[13] The patient showed OCA with generalized hypopigmentation, nystagmus, iris transillumination, and retinal hypopigmentation; respiratory distress requiring a 3 week admission to a neonatal intensive-care unit for respiratory support; and platelet electron microscopy showing absent platelet delta granules.[13]

Recombinant factor VIIa (rFVIIa) is useful for dangerous bleeding such as refractory menorrhagia.[19] Progressive HPS-1 pulmonary fibrosis is effectively treated by pirfenidone, a small molecule that inhibits TGF-beta-mediated fibroblast proliferation and collagen synthesis *in vitro*.[20] Infliximab is effective for granulomatous colitis in HPS patients.[21] The efficacy of infliximab suggests that TNF-α plays a pivotal role in the pathogenesis.[21]

3. The mice and rat models of HPS

Mice models of HPS can be grouped into BLOC-3 (*pale ear*[22, 23] and *light ear*[9]), BLOC-2 (*cocoa*[24], *ruby-eye-2*[10] and *ruby-eye*[10]), BLOC-1 (*sandy*[11], *reduced pigmentation*[25], *pallid*[26], *cappuccino*[27] and *muted*[28]), AP-3 (*pearl*[29] and *mocha*[30]), class C VPS (*buff*[31]), RABGGT (*gunmetal*[32]), and others (*misty*[33] and *subtle gray*[34]) (**Table 1**). Two rat models of HPS, Fawn-Hooded Rat and Tester-Moriyama Rat, are genetically identical with no expression of *RAB38*.[35]

Gautam *et al.* contacted mutant mice doubly or triply deficient in protein subunits of the various BLOC complexes and/or the AP-3 adaptor complex and tested for viability and for abnormalities of lysosome-related organelles (LROs) including melanosomes, lamellar bodies of lung type II cells and platelet dense granules.[36] They showed that double and triple mutant HPS mice provide unique and practical experimental advantages in the study of LROs.[36] Long-Evans Cinnamon rats with a point mutation in the initiation codon of Rab38 small GTPase are investigated for the pathogenesis of interstitial pneumonia via aberrant lung surfactant secretion.[37] Thus, mice and rat models are indispensable for recognizing the molecular function in LROs and the pathogenesis of HPS.

4. The molecular functions

The complexes involving in the pathogenesis of HPS are BLOC-3, BLOC-2, BLOC-1, AP-3 adaptor complex, and class C VPS. BLOC-3 is composed of HPS1/pale ear and HPS4/light ear.[38-40] BLOC-2 conprises HPS3/cocoa, HPS5/ruby-eye-2 and HPS6/ruby-eye.[10, 41] BLOC-1 is constructed by proteins of HPS7/DTNBP1/sandy, HPS8/BLOC1S3/reduced pigmentation/ BLOS3, cappuccino, muted, pallid, BLOS1, BLOS2 and snapin.[42, 43] AP-3 (subunits δ/mocha, β3/HPS2/ AP3B1/pearl, μ3, σ3) is one of the family of heterotetrameric clathrin adaptors.[44] The class C VPS is composed of VPS11, VPS16, VPS18, and VPS33/buff.[45]

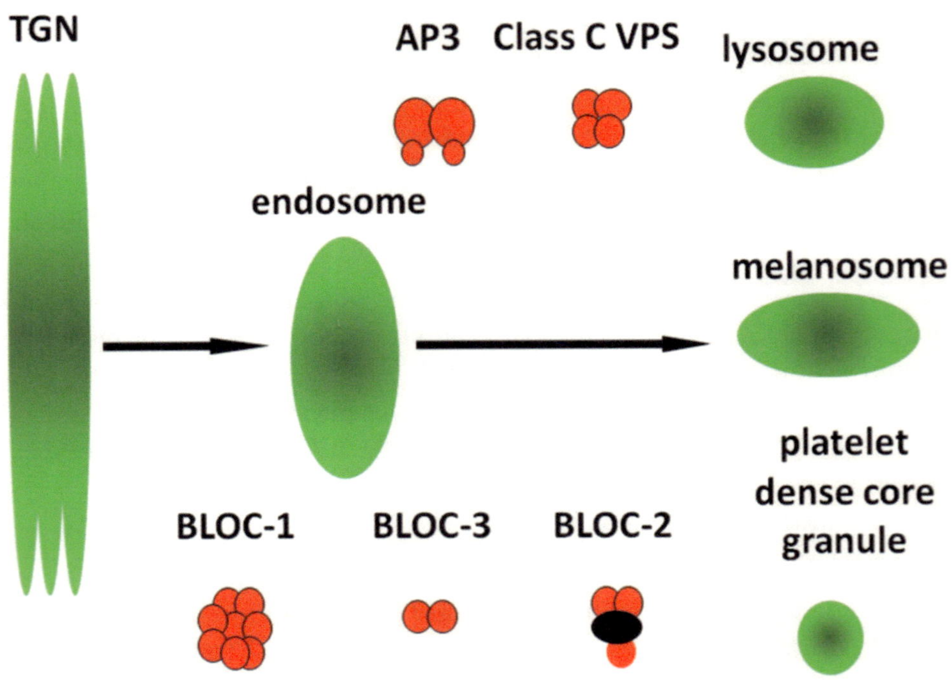

Figure 1. BLOC-1, -2, -3, AP-3 and class C VPS complexes involve in membrane trafficking from endosomes to lysosomes and lysosome-related organelles, melanosomes and dense core granules in platelets.

Adaptor protein complexes are composed of heterotetramers (two large subunits, a medium-sized subunit and a small subunit) and sort cargo into vesicles for transport from one membrane compartment of the cell to another.[46] AP-3 traffics cargo from tubular endosomes to late endosomes, lysosomes, and related organelles via the bound to BLOC-1, vimentin, clathrin and others.[46, 47]

The class C VPS core complex (VPS33A/B, VPS11, VPS16 and VPS18) is essential for late endosome and lysosome assembly and for numerous endolysosomal trafficking pathways.[48] Two class C VPC complexes, homotypic fusion and protein sorting (HOPS) and class C core vacuole/endosome tethering (CORVET), incorporate diverse biochemical functions: they tether membranes, stimulate Rab nucleotide exchange, guide SNARE assembly to drive membrane fusion, and possibly act as ubiquitin ligases.[48]

BLOC-1 functions in selective cargo exit from early endosomes toward lysosomes and lysosome-related organelles such as melanosomes and BLOC-2 act sequentially in the same pathway.[49] Melanosome maturation requires at least two cargo transport pathways directly from early endosomes to melanosomes, one pathway mediated by AP-3 and one pathway mediated by BLOC-1 and BLOC-2.[49] BLOC-3 is constructed by HPS1 and HPS4 heterodimers.[50] BLOC-3 interacts with the GTP-bound form of the endosomal GTPase, Rab9. BLOC-3 might function as a Rab9 effector in the biogenesis of lysosome-related organelles.[50]

5. Conclusion

Now, HPS is a representative disorder of aberrant membrane trafficking. HPS genes have been identified with mice models. The function of encoded proteins has been accompanied with cell biology in yeast, worm, fly and animal models. Membrane trafficking is crucial for cells to survive and play their active functions. Further emerging investigation will reveal more precise pathogenesis in HPS.

Aberrations

biogenesis of lysosome related organelle complex (BLOC)-1, -2, -3

adaptor protein complex 3 (AP3)

vacuolar protein sorting (VPS)

Rab geranylgeranyl transferase (RABGGT)

homotypic fusion and protein sorting (HOPS)

class C core vacuole/endosome tethering (CORVET)

Author details

Naoki Oiso and Akira Kawada
Departments of Dermatology, Kinki University Faculty of Medicine, Osaka-Sayama, Osaka, Japan

6. References

[1] Hermansky F, Pudlak P. Albinism associated with hemorrhagic diathesis and unusual pigmented reticular cells in the bone marrow: report of two cases with histochemical studies. *Blood* 1959; 14: 162-9.

[2] Oh J, Ho L, Ala-Mello S, *et al*. Mutation analysis of patients with Hermansky-Pudlak syndrome: a frameshift hot spot in the HPS gene and apparent locus heterogeneity. *Am J Hum Genet* 1998; 62: 593-598.

[3] Li W, Rusiniak ME, Chintala S, *et al*. Murine Hermansky-Pudlak syndrome genes: regulators of lysosome-related organelles. *Bioessays* 2004; 26: 616-28.

[4] Di Pietro SM, Dell'Angelica EC. The cell biology of Hermansky-Pudlak syndrome: recent advances. *Traffic* 2005; 6: 525-33.

[5] Huizing M, Helip-Wooley A, Westbroek W, *et al.* Disorders of lysosome-related organelle biogenesis: clinical and molecular genetics. *Annu Rev Genomics Hum Genet* 2008; 9: 359-86.

[6] Oh J*, Bailin T*, Fukai K*, Feng GH*, *et al* (*co-first author). Positional cloning of a gene for Hermansky-Pudlak syndrome, a disorder of cytoplasmic organelles. *Nat Genet* 1996; 14: 300-6.

[7] Dell'Angelica EC, Shotelersuk V, Aguilar RC, *et al.* Altered trafficking of lysosomal proteins in Hermansky-Pudlak syndrome due to mutations in the beta 3A subunit of the AP-3 adaptor. *Mol Cell* 1999; 3: 11-21.

[8] Anikster Y, Huizing M, White J, *et al.* Mutation of a new gene causes a unique form of Hermansky-Pudlak syndrome in a genetic isolate of central Puerto Rico. *Nat Genet* 2001; 28: 376-80.

[9] Suzuki T, Li W, Zhang Q, *et al.* Hermansky-Pudlak syndrome is caused by mutations in HPS4, the human homolog of the mouse light-ear gene. *Nat Genet* 2002; 30: 321-4.

[10] Zhang Q*, Zhao B*, Li W*, Oiso N*, *et al* (*co-first author). Ru2 and Ru encode mouse orthologs of the genes mutated in human Hermansky-Pudlak syndrome types 5 and 6. *Nat Genet* 2003; 33: 145-53.

[11] Li W*, Zhang Q*, Oiso N*, *et al* (*co-first author). Hermansky-Pudlak syndrome type 7 (HPS-7) results from mutant dysbindin, a member of the biogenesis of lysosome-related organelles complex 1 (BLOC-1). *Nat Genet* 2003; 35: 84-9.

[12] Morgan NV, Pasha S, Johnson CA, *et al.* A germline mutation in BLOC1S3/reduced pigmentation causes a novel variant of Hermansky-Pudlak syndrome (HPS8). *Am J Hum Genet* 2006; 78: 160-6.

[13] Cullinane AR, Curry JA, Carmona-Rivera C, *et al.* A BLOC-1 mutation screen reveals that PLDN is mutated in Hermansky-Pudlak Syndrome type 9. *Am J Hum Genet* 2011; 88: 778-87.

[14] Gochuico BR, Huizing M, Golas GA, *et al.* Interstitial lung disease and pulmonary fibrosis in Hermansky-Pudlak syndrome type 2, an adaptor protein-3 complex disease. *Mol Med* 2012; 18: 56-64.

[15] Huizing M, Anikster Y, Fitzpatrick DL, *et al.* Hermansky-Pudlak syndrome type 3 in Ashkenazi Jews and other non-Puerto Rican patients with hypopigmentation and platelet storage-pool deficiency. *Am J Hum Genet* 2001; 69: 1022-32.

[16] Huizing M, Hess R, Dorward H, *et al.* Cellular, molecular and clinical characterization of patients with Hermansky-Pudlak syndrome type 5. *Traffic* 2004; 5: 711-22.

[17] Huizing M, Pederson B, Hess RA, *et al.* Clinical and cellular characterisation of Hermansky-Pudlak syndrome type 6. *J Med Genet* 2009; 46: 803-10.

[18] Cullinane AR, Curry JA, Golas G, *et al.* A BLOC-1 mutation screen reveals a novel BLOC1S3 mutation in Hermansky-Pudlak Syndrome type 8. *Pigment Cell Melanoma Res* 2012; 25: 584-91.

[19] Lohse J, Gehrisch S, Tauer JT, *et al.* Therapy refractory menorrhagia as first manifestation of Hermansky-Pudlak syndrome. *Hamostaseologie* 2011; 31 Suppl 1: S61-3.

[20] O'Brien K, Troendle J, Gochuico BR, *et al*. Pirfenidone for the treatment of Hermansky-Pudlak syndrome pulmonary fibrosis. *Mol Genet Metab* 2011; 103: 128-34.

[21] Grucela AL, Patel P, Goldstein E, *et al*. Granulomatous enterocolitis associated with Hermansky-Pudlak syndrome. *Am J Gastroenterol* 2006; 101: 2090-5.

[22] Gardner JM, Wildenberg SC, Keiper NM, *et al*. The mouse pale ear (ep) mutation is the homologue of human Hermansky-Pudlak syndrome. *Proc Natl Acad Sci U S A* 1997; 94: 9238-43.

[23] Feng GH, Bailin T, Oh J, *et al*. Mouse pale ear (*ep*) is homologous to human Hermansky-Pudlak syndrome and contains a rare 'AT-AC' intron. *Hum Mol Genet* 1997; 6: 793-7.

[24] Suzuki T*, Li W*, Zhang Q, *et al* (*co-first author). The gene mutated in cocoa mice, carrying a defect of organelle biogenesis, is a homologue of the human Hermansky-Pudlak syndrome-3 gene. *Genomics* 2001; 78: 30-7.

[25] Gwynn B, Martina JA, Bonifacino JS, *et al*. Reduced pigmentation (rp), a mouse model of Hermansky-Pudlak syndrome, encodes a novel component of the BLOC-1 complex. *Blood* 2004; 104: 3181-9.

[26] Huang L, Kuo YM, Gitschier J, *et al*. The pallid gene encodes a novel, syntaxin 13-interacting protein involved in platelet storage pool deficiency. *Nat Genet* 1999; 23: 329-32.

[27] Cicciotte SC, Gwynn B, Moriyaka K, *et al*. Cappuccino, a mouse model of Hermansky-Pudlak syndrome, encodes a novel protein that is part of the pallidin-muted complex (BLOC-1). *Blood* 2003; 101: 4402-7.

[28] Zhang Q*, Li W*, Novak EK, *et al* (*co-first author). The gene for the muted (mu) mouse, a model for Hermansky-Pudlak syndrome, defines a novel protein which regulates vesicle trafficking. *Hum Mol Genet* 2002; 11: 697-706.

[29] Feng L*, Seymour AB*, Jiang S, *et al* (*co-first author). The beta3A subunit gene (Ap3b1) of the AP-3 adaptor complex is altered in the mouse hypopigmentation mutant pearl, a model for Hermansky-Pudlak syndrome and night blindness. *Hum Mol Genet* 1999; 8: 323-30.

[30] Kantheti P, Qiao X, Diaz ME, *et al*. Mutation in AP-3 delta in the mocha mouse links endosomal transport to storage deficiency in platelets, melanosomes, and synaptic vesicles. *Neuron* 1998; 21: 111-22.

[31] Suzuki T*, Oiso N*, Gautam R*, *et al* (co-first author). The mouse organellar biogenesis mutant buff results from a mutation in Vps33a, a homologue of yeast vps33 and Drosophila carnation. *Proc Natl Acad Sci U S A* 2003; 100: 1146-50.

[32] Detter JC, Zhang Q, Mules EH, *et al*. Rab geranylgeranyl transferase alpha mutation in the gunmetal mouse reduces Rab prenylation and platelet synthesis. *Proc Natl Acad Sci U S A* 2000; 97: 4144-9.

[33] Blasius AL, Brandl K, Crozat K, *et al*. Mice with mutations of Dock7 have generalized hypopigmentation and white-spotting but show normal neurological function. *Proc Natl Acad Sci U S A* 2009; 106: 2706-11.

[34] Chintala S, Li W, Lamoreux ML, *et al*. Slc7a11 gene controls production of pheomelanin pigment and proliferation of cultured cells. *Proc Natl Acad Sci USA* 2005; 102: 10964-9.

[35] Oiso N, Riddle SR, Serikawa T, *et al.* The rat Ruby (R) locus is Rab38: identical mutations in Fawn-hooded and Tester-Moriyama rats derived from an ancestral Long Evans rat sub-strain. *Mamm Genome* 2004; 15: 307-14.
[36] Gautam R, Novak EK, Tan J, *et al.* Interaction of Hermansky-Pudlak Syndrome genes in the regulation of lysosome-related organelles. *Traffic* 2006; 7: 779-92.
[37] Osanai K, Higuchi J, Oikawa R, *et al.* Altered lung surfactant system in a Rab38-deficient rat model of Hermansky-Pudlak syndrome. *Am J Physiol Lung Cell Mol Physiol* 2010; 298: L243-51.
[38] Chiang PW, Oiso N, Gautam R, *et al.* The Hermansky-Pudlak syndrome 1 (HPS1) and HPS4 proteins are components of two complexes, BLOC-3 and BLOC-4, involved in the biogenesis of lysosome-related organelles. *J Biol Chem* 2003; 278: 20332-7.
[39] Martina JA, Moriyama K, Bonifacino JS. BLOC-3, a protein complex containing the Hermansky-Pudlak syndrome gene products HPS1 and HPS4. *J Biol Chem* 2003; 278: 29376-84.
[40] Nazarian R, Falcon-Perez JM, Dell'angelica EC. Biogenesis of lysosome-related organelles complex 3 (BLOC-3): a complex containing the Hermansky-Pudlak syndrome (HPS) proteins HPS1 and HPS4. *Proc Natl Acad Sci U S A* 2003; 100: 8770-5.
[41] Gautam R, Chintala S, Li W, *et al.* The Hermansky-Pudlak syndrome 3 (cocoa) protein is a component of the biogenesis of lysosome-related organelles complex-2 (BLOC-2). *J Biol Chem* 2004; 279: 12935-42.
[42] Falcon-Perez JM, Starcevic M, Gautam R, *et al.* BLOC-1, a novel complex containing the pallidin and muted proteins involved in the biogenesis of melanosomes and platelet-dense granules. *J Biol Chem* 2002; 277: 28191-9.
[43] Starcevic M, Dell'angelica EC. Identification of snapin and three novel proteins (BLOS1, BLOS2, and BLOS3/reduced pigmentation) as subunits of biogenesis of lysosome-related organelles complex-1 (BLOC-1). *J Biol Chem* 2004; 279: 28393-401.
[44] Simpson F, Bright NA, West MA, *et al.* A novel adaptor-related protein complex. *J Cell Biol* 1996; 133: 749-60.
[45] Sato TK, Rehling P, Peterson MR, *et al.* Class C Vps protein complex regulates vacuolar SNARE pairing and is required for vesicle docking/fusion. *Mol Cell* 2000; 6: 661-71.
[46] Hirst J, Barlow LD, Francisco GC, *et al.* The fifth adaptor protein complex. *PLoS Biol* 2011; 9: e1001170.
[47] Newell-Litwa K, Seong E, Burmeister M, *et al.* Neuronal and non-neuronal functions of the AP-3 sorting machinery. *J Cell Sci* 2007; 120: 531-41.
[48] Nickerson DP, Brett CL, Merz AJ. Vps-C complexes: gatekeepers of endolysosomal traffic. *Curr Opin Cell Biol* 2009; 21: 543-51.
[49] Setty SR, Tenza D, Truschel ST, *et al.* BLOC-1 is required for cargo-specific sorting from vacuolar early endosomes toward lysosome-related organelles. *Mol Biol Cell* 2007; 18: 768-80.
[50] Kloer DP, Rojas R, Ivan V, *et al.* Assembly of the biogenesis of lysosome-related organelles complex-3 (BLOC-3) and its interaction with Rab9. *J Biol Chem* 2010; 285: 7794-804.

Chapter 9

Dyschromatosis Symmetrica Hereditaria and RNA Editing Enzyme

Michihiro Kono and Masashi Akiyama

Additional information is available at the end of the chapter

http://dx.doi.org/10.5772/55203

1. Introduction

Dyschromatosis symmetrica hereditaria (DSH) is a highly penetrant autosomal-dominant skin disease. It is characterized by a mixture of hyper- and hypo-pigmented macules on the dorsal aspects of the hands and feet (Figure 1). The disorder typically has its onset during infancy or early childhood, stops spreading before adolescence and lasts for life. It was clarified in 2003 that a heterozygous mutation in the adenosine deaminase acting on RNA1 gene (*ADAR1*) causes DSH [1].

The ADAR1 protein catalyzes the deamination of adenosine to inosine in double-stranded RNA [2, 3]. This modification is called RNA editing, more specifically A-I editing (Figure 2).

RNA editing is a post-transcriptional modification, and A-I editing is widely conserved in species ranging from roundworm to mammals. A-I editing had been considered a rare phenomenon in the coding region and this editing is known to create alterations of the codon or alternative splice sites that lead to different proteins in the target substrate. Representative substrate genes are the ionotropic AMPA glutamate receptor subunit 2 [4] and the 5-HT2c serotonin receptor [5], which are both expressed in the brain and are associated with the some neurologic diseases [6].

However, the substrate gene for ADAR1 in the skin and the pathogenic mechanisms whereby mutation in *ADAR1* causes DSH remain unknown.

This chapter addresses DSH. First, we introduce the clinical and pathological features of DSH. Next, we introduce how *ADAR1* was identified as the causative gene of DSH. I mention ADAR1 and A-I editing, ADAR1 isoforms and DSH, the absence of a correlation between the DSH phenotype and mutation in *ADAR1*, and murine models of DSH.

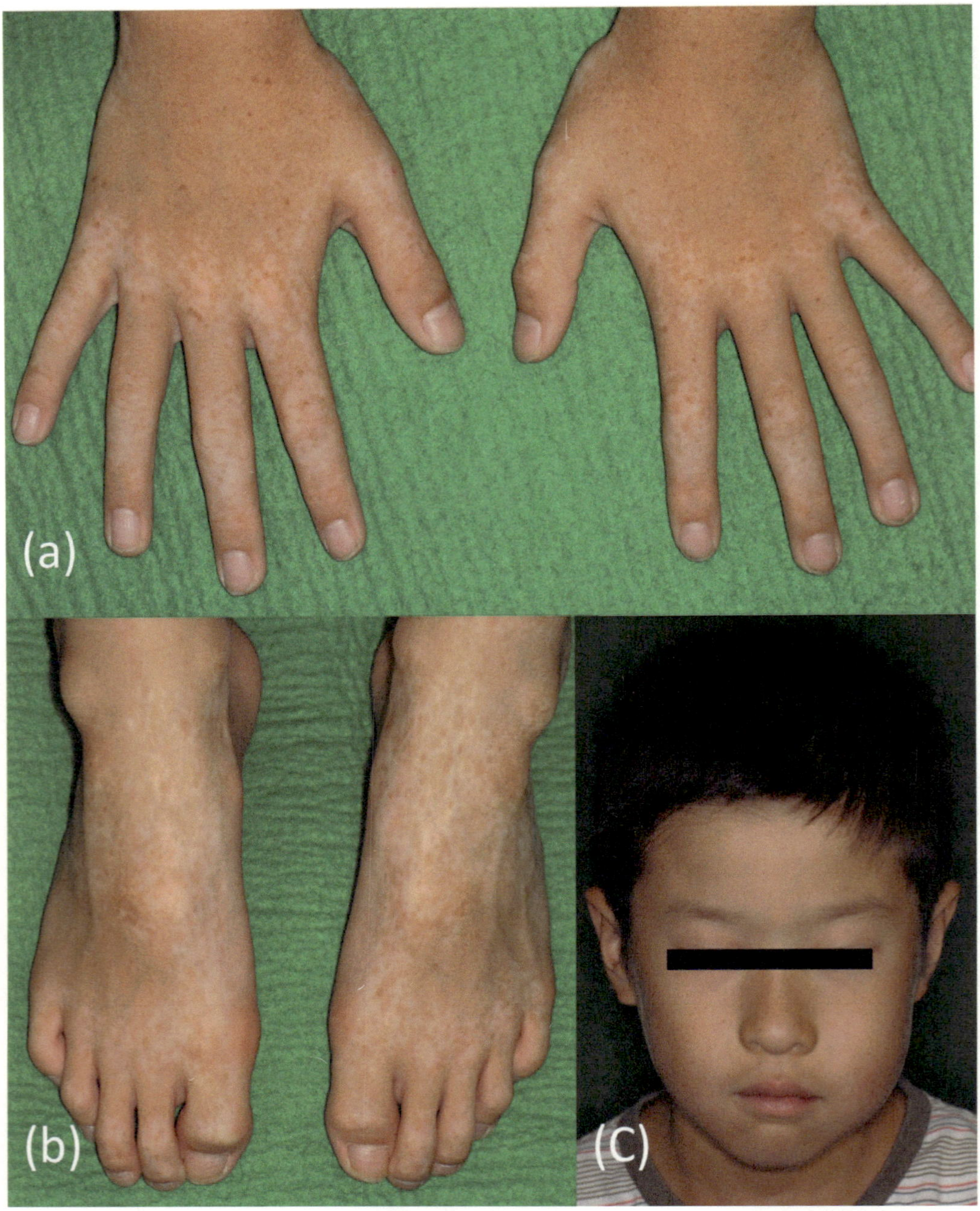

Figure 1. Clinical features of dyschromatosis symmetrica hereditaria. The patient is an 8-year-old boy. His hands and feet show hyper- and hypopigmented macules (a, b). On the face, he has small freckle-like, light-brown macules (c).

2. DSH, ADAR1 and RNA editing

2.1. Epidemiology and clinical features of DSH

Dyschromatosis symmetrica hereditaria (DSH; OMIM#127400; also called reticulate acropigmentation of Dohi) is an autosomal-dominant pigmentary genodermatosis with almost full penetrance. DSH was first described by Toyama [7, 8].

Clinically, the disorder is characterized by areas several millimeters in diameter of mixed hypopigmented and hyperpigmented macules distributed predominantly on the dorsal aspects of the hands and feet but sometimes extending to the dorsal aspects of the limbs (Figure 1). The lesions on the face are described as freckle-like macules with no hypopigmentation [9, 10]; some cases have been reported in which mixed areas of hypopigmented and hyperpigmented macules on the cheek were similar to those on the hands and feet [11]. Patients who have strong skin manifestations on the limbs also tend to have lesions on face. The skin lesions do not show telangiectasia, atrophy or scaling. Skin manifestations are not observed on the palm, sole or mucosa.

DSH has been reported mainly from Japan and China; however, patients in South Korea [12], Taiwan [13], Thailand [11], India [14], Turkey [15] and Europe [16, 17] and patients of Hispanic ethnicity [18] have been reported.

The disorder typically develops during infancy or early childhood [19]. Lesions first appear before the age of 6 years in 73% of cases, and the first appearance is usually on the limbs (83%) [20], particularly the hands and feet. This point can be useful in differentiating the disorder from dyschromatosis universalis symmetrica (DUH). The macules enlarge progressively [16], stop spreading before adolescence and last for life [19, 21]. The onset of lesions during adolescence has been reported in some patients [22].

The skin findings are more pronounced after sun exposure, although patients do not show photosensitivity [10, 20]. This differentiates the disorder from xeroderma pigmentosum (XP).

Interfamilial and intrafamilial variation has been reported. The clinical features are not always similar among patients in a pedigree [23]. We have encountered a family in which the patient has only faint hypopigmented macules on the backs of the fingers and the patient's children have mixtures of hyper- and hypopigmented macules in all the limbs.

The characteristic clinical features of typical DSH can be clearly differentially diagnosed from similar hereditary pigmentary disorders as follows [9]. Acropigmentatio reticularis (Kitamura) (ARK) is characterized by atrophic pigmented macules on the dorsum of the hands and feet, and palmoplantar pits and pigmentation. It is autosomal dominant, as is DSH.

DUH shows hypo- and hyper-pigmented macules that are similar to those of DSH on the trunk as well as the extremities. It has been reported to be autosomal dominant and autosomal recessive.

It had been though that those two diseases were related to DSH. However, when mutation of the *ADAR1* gene was identified as causing DSH, it was clarified that the two diseases are genetically distinct from DSH, because patients with ARK and DUH do not have that mutation [9].

Mild cases or the early stages of child DSH are sometimes difficult to differentiate from xeroderma pigmentosum (XP) [24]. In such cases, the diagnosis of XP can usually be obtained by following up on skin lesions such as xerosis, atrophy, telangiectasia and skin tumors of sun-exposed areas as they grow up, photosensitivity test, and ultimately gene analysis [24, 25].

2.2. Histopathology of DSH

Histological studies have showed increased melanin pigmentation in the basal layer of hyperpigmented lesions, along with pigmentary incontinence and largely absent melanin in the hypopigmented macule [13, 23].

According to precise histochemical studies, Masson-Fontana stain reveals a remarkable decrease or total absence of melanin in the hypochromic-achromic epidermis [13, 23]. Split-dopa preparations were reported to show an obvious decrease in melanocyte number in the hypomelanotic area (45-167 cells/mm^2) and the surrounding pigmented skin (119-204 cells/mm^2), as compared with the 16 normal control persons (1,217+/-282 cells/mm^2 on the dorsal hands and 821-1,154 cells/mm^2 on the dorsal feet) [13]. There was an increase in melanocyte size but not number in the hyperchromic area, and the dendrites were very elongated and numerous, suggesting that melanosome transfer from melanocytes to keratinocytes was active [13]. Another study also indicated a lower density of dopa-positive melanocytes in the hypo-pigmented macules of DSH patients than in normal skin at same site from normal pigmented controls [26]. Electron microscopy showed melanocytic abnormalities in the hypomelanotic skin, i.e., a numerical decrease, fatty degeneration, swollen mitochondria, vacuolization of the cytoplasm, large cytoplasmic vacuole formation and condensed irregularly shaped nuclei [13, 23]. The keratinocytes located in the vicinity of the melanocytes contained few melanosomes. In some keratinocytes, the melanosome complex containing more than 15 melanosomes were recognized [13]. The hyperpigmented area showed a lot of slight larger melanosomes in the melanocytes, and the adjacent keratinocytes showed many singly dispersed melanosomes [13]. The aggregated melanosome were also found in the keratinocyte in hyperpigmented macules [23]. In the hyperpigmented macules, the number of melanosomes in the melanocytes was somewhat smaller than in adjacent keratinocytes, which suggests that the melanosome transfer from melanocytes to keratinocytes is more active than melanosome production in the melanocyte [23].

2.3. Identifying the causative gene of DSH

In 2003, Miyamura et al. determined that a heterozygous mutation of the adenosine deaminase acting on RNA1 gene (*ADAR1*) caused DSH [1]. As there was no clue to predict the pathogenesis of DSH at that time, they used a technique called positional cloning to identify the causative gene. Positional cloning locates the position of a disease-associated gene along the chromosome by a collection of methods including linkage analysis, haplotype analysis, genomic mapping and sequencing. This approach works even when little or no information is available about the biochemical basis of the disease.

In identifying the causative gene of DSH [1], whole-genome-wide scan (linkage analysis) using 343 microsatellite markers in three pedigrees of DSH (88 people, including 41 patients) was done at first. The results of linkage analysis indicated that the DSH locus was on the long arm of chromosome 1. Next, to narrow the interval of the region containing the DSH locus, haplotype analysis was carried out, and the results suggested that the DSH gene lay between two microsatellite markers, D1S2715 and D1S2777. Haplotype analysis using novel single-nucleotide polymorphisms showed a final DSH genetic interval of approximately 500 kbp. There were 9 genes in this interval, including the *ADAR1* gene. Finally, it was clarified that all of the patients with DSH had mutations in the *ADAR1* gene. Thus it was concluded that the *ADAR1* gene was the causative gene of DSH [1].

The ADAR1 protein catalyzes the deamination of adenosine to inosine in double-stranded RNA [2, 3]. ADAR1 is in the ADAR protein family, which includes ADAR1 [6], ADAR2 [27] and ADAR3 [28]. As RNA editing enzymes, all ADAR family members contain several double-stranded RNA-binding domains (dsRBDs) and a conserved catalytic deaminase domain in the C-terminal region [29]. Differences in the number and spacing of the dsRBDs, nuclear localization signals and the presence of additional domains create the variants (Figure 2A).

The *ADAR1* gene spans 30 kbp and contains 15 exons. The encoded 1226 amino acid protein includes three dsRBDs and one dsRNA adenosine deaminase catalytic domain [30].

ADAR1 has two isoforms of different sizes: interferon-inducible ADAR1-p150 (150kDa) and constitutively expressed ADAR1-p110 (110kDa) (Figure 2B) [30]. Both contain three dsRBDs, but they differ in that the p150 variant contains two Z-DNA binding domains and a nuclear export signal, whereas the p110 variant contains only a single Z-DNA binding domain and no export signal. Consequently, ADAR1-p110 localizes mainly to the nucleus, whereas ADAR1-p150 is found in both the cytoplasm and the nucleus. Resulting from alternative promoters, the two variants may play different cellular roles. Although the ADAR1-p110 promoter is constitutively active, the ADAR1-p150 promoter is interferon-inducible, suggesting a role in response to cellular stresses such as viral infection [31].

ADAR1 catalyzes the deamination of adenosine to inosine in double-stranded RNA substrates in the step of post-transcription processing [2] (Figure 3). Inosine acts as guanine during translation, which results in codon alterations or alternative splicing sites [32] and thus leads to functional changes in proteins. It is expressed ubiquitously, including in the skin [29], but only a few known target genes for ADAR1 are expressed in specific tissues, including ionotropic glutamate receptor [33] [34] and the serotonin receptor 2C subtype in the brain [5], and hepatitis δ virus antigen in the liver [35]. Fifteen sites of amino acid substitution by A-I editing have been identified to date [36]. The substrate gene edited by

ADAR1 in the skin is still unknown, and it remains to clarify how ADAR1 causes DSH. The structure and function of ADAR1 are detailed later.

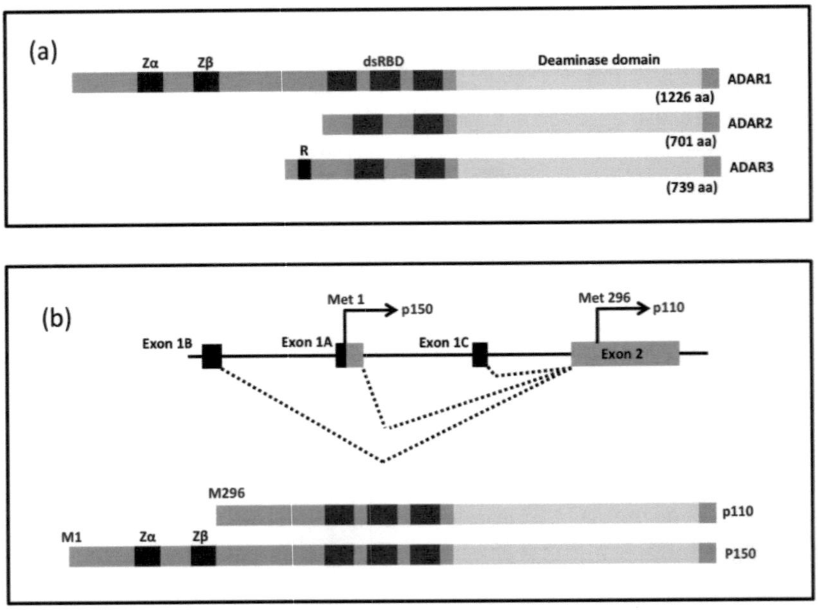

Figure 2. The human ADAR gene family. (a) The structure of the human ADAR gene family: ADAR1, ADAR2 and ADAR3. The dsRNA binding domains (dsRBDs) and the deaminase domain exist in all three ADARs. Two Z-DNA binding domains (Zα and Zβ) exist in ADAR1. ADAR3 includes an arginine-rich domain (the R-domain) and an ssRNA binding domain, but the function of those two domains is still unknown. (b) Two isoforms of ADAR1. Exon 1A, exon 1B and exon1C are spliced to exon 2 at precisely the same junction. Exon1A contains the Met initiation codon for the p150 isoform (1226 aa) and follows the interferon-inducible promoter. Exon 1B and exon1C do not contain an AUG initiation codon. Those exons follow a constitutive promoter. The second AUG at 296aa from the first AUG located in exon 2 initiates translation of the other isoform, p110, which is constitutively expressed.

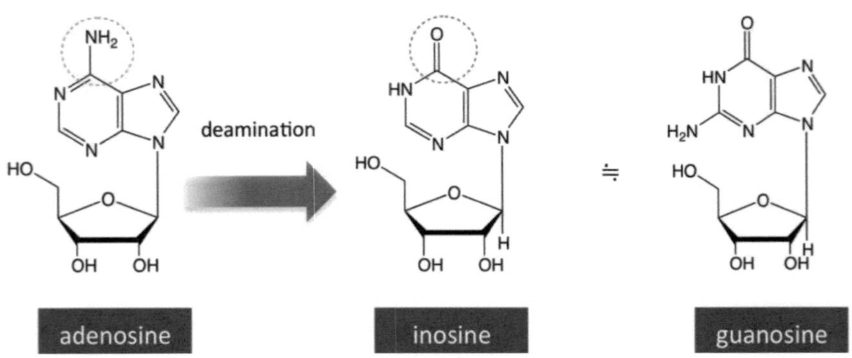

Figure 3. Adenosine deamination by ADARs. ADARs convert adenosines to inosines of double-stranded RNA by catalyzing a hydrolytic deamination at C6 of the adenine base. This modification is called RNA editing, more specifically, A-I editing. Inosine is recognized as guanosine at translation, and this editing produces codon change. Also, it creates alternative splice sites. These both lead to different proteins in the target substrate. Recently a lot of non-coding RNA has also been found to be substrates of ADARs.

2.4. Gene analysis of the *ADAR1* in DSH patients

Since identification of the *ADAR1* gene, more than 115 mutations in the gene have been reported in patients with DSH [37]. The distribution of mutations shows no hotspots, with the mutations distributed equally in coding regions. Every type of mutation—nonsense, missense, insertion, deletion and splice-site—has been identified in the gene. No founder effect has been recognized [9]. Major part of mutations have been identified in Japanese and Chinese, and some reports show mutations in *ADAR1* for DSH patients of other races. Characteristically, all the missense mutations are in the adenosine deaminase catalytic domain. Thus it is thought that this domain is a very critical one. Functional analysis of the adenosine deaminase catalytic domain has indicated different mutant ADAR1 enzymes in which the missense mutation on the deaminase domain has caused complete abolishment of the deaminase activity, though there were some exceptions [38]. Notably, mutations that leave some enzyme activity intact are not found in DSH patients. The result of this experiment does not mean that DSH patient looses ADAR1 activity completely because DSH is autosomal dominant and half of ADAR1 protein are intact.

The two mutations p.Q102fs and p.H216fs [9, 39] that were found in the *ADAR1* gene of DSH patients were previously reported, and they are on the 5' side upstream of codon 296 in exon 2, which is the translation initiation codon for hADAR1-p110 (Fig. 2B). Therefore, it is possible that they cause a frameshift change in the synthesis of hADAR1-p150 but have no influence on that of ADAR1-p110. This suggests that only the p150 protein and the interferon-inducible (IFN) mechanism are responsible for the etiology of DSH.

2.5. Homodimerization of ADAR1

Homodimerization was demonstrated to be essential for the enzyme activity of ADAR1 [40]. Having one monomer defective for the deaminase domain (E396A) halves the dimer function. Taken together, these data indicate that a deaminase mutant chimeric dimer (E396A/WT) is able to bind dsRNA but that only one functional active site is formed and the result is, therefore, only partial activity [40]. This result may indicate that ADAR1 mutation in the deaminase domain generates haploinsufficiency. However, site-selective RNA editing activity of $5HT_{2C}R$ RNA by heterodimer was found to be decreased to 30% [40]. These results may indicate a complex effect at each site by this enzyme.

In contrast, the A-I editing activity of the dsRNA binding mutant chimeric dimer (Mut/WT) is completely lost [41]. This is because of the defective dsRBDs of one monomer, and it suggests that cooperative interactions of functional dsRBDs in both ADAR dimer subunits are required for dsRNA binding. When one monomer in the dimer complex is unable to bind the dsRNA, then the dimer complex is excluded from binding the substrate. It shows activity. As previously indicated, in DSH patients, a disproportionately high number of mutations are identified in the deaminase domain relative to the dsRBDs of ADAR1. It may be that mutations identified in the deaminase domain are less severe, because the chimeric dimers that are expected to form still retain some editing activity [41].

The likely ratio of monomer subunits in a dimer is 1:2:1 for (WT/WT), (Mut/WT) and (Mut/Mut), suggesting that a heterozygous deaminase mutation would not have as strong an effect due to the dimer's ability to maintain partial activity. In contrast, mutations are rarely found in the dsRBDs, because these alterations would have a more dominant effect when paired with a wild-type partner, thus greatly reducing ADAR function. Under this assumption, the reduced activity for ADAR could be as low as one-quarter with only (WT/WT) dimers having editing activity, and this may be below a threshold for survival and may possibly be selected out naturally during development. ADAR dimerization can be a potential source of modulation for RNA editing activity, and these ADAR (EAA) mutants may prove interesting for future studies *in vivo* [41]. So, DSH can be regarded as being induced by haploinsufficiency of ADAR1. Three DSH cases with neurological complications have been reported [16, 21, 42]. Two of these cases were confirmed by gene analysis [21, 42], and the *ADAR1* gene mutation that they have is common and is thought to show a dominant negative effect. The next section describes those cases.

2.6. Neurological complications

In 1994, Patrizi *et al.* reported a 9-year-old Caucasian girl who developed DSH at the age of 2 years and torsion dystonia at the age of 7 years [16]. Her clinical symptoms were very similar to the latter 2 cases, but mental deterioration and brain calcification were not described in their report [16]. The causative gene of DSH had not been clarified, and no information on *ADAR1* gene analysis of the patient was reported.

Tojo *et al.* reported a 27-year-old Japanese woman who had dystonia, mental deterioration, brain calcification and DSH with a p.G1007R mutation of the *ADAR* gene [42]. Kondo *et al.* reported an 11-year-old Japanese boy who also had mental deterioration, brain calcification and dystonia and DSH with a p.G1007R mutation of the *ADAR* gene [21]. It is noteworthy that the two patients had the same *ADAR1* mutation, p.G1007R, and it suggests that this mutation probably influences the development of neurological symptoms [21].

On the basis of the known crystal structure [43], it was predicted that ADAR1 G1007R would introduce an additional positively charged arginine residue on the RNA-binding face of the deaminase domain very close to the active site [44]. In fact, the ADAR1 G1007R mutant has efficient RNA-binding ability, similar in level to that of wild-type ADAR1, but it does not edit dsRNA; however, other mutant ADAR1 partially edit. So, the dominant negative effect gives these additional neurological symptoms of DSH [44, 45].

The ionotropic glutamate receptor [33, 34] is a known target gene for ADAR1. Glutamate receptors are expressed at high levels in the brain, including in the basal ganglia [46], and glutamatergic overactivity has been suggested to contribute to the occurrence of dystonia [47, 48]. ADAR1 catalyzes RNA editing at the Q/R sites of the glutamate receptor subunits GluR5 and GluR6, and reduces the Ca^{2+} permeability of glutamate receptors [49]. Therefore, mutation in *ADAR1* could reduce the efficiency of RNA editing at the Q/R sites of GluR5 and GluR6, inducing glutamatergic overactivity.

Furthermore, increased Ca^{2+} influx through glutamate receptors is known to be toxic to neurons, and that toxicity may induce various neurological abnormalities [50]. Increases in intracellular Ca^{2+} levels have also been reported to be the underlying mechanism of tissue calcification [51]. Therefore, mutations in *ADAR1* could conceivably cause neurological dysfunction, such as dystonia and mental deterioration, by means of brain calcification [51], but only the p.G1007R mutation has so far been suggested to be related to such symptoms, and the pathomechanism remains unknown.

The patient's mother had the same mutation in p.G1007R as her son, but she showed no neurological problems, which suggests that some unknown mechanism is involved in the development of dystonia, mental deterioration and brain calcification [52]. It will be necessary to observe whether she develops neurological symptoms later. This mechanism, as well as the unknown molecular pathogenesis of the skin lesion, should be clarified.

2.7. More ADAR functions than A-I editing of the coding region of mRNA

Only a few sites of A-I editing by ADAR1 had been found in the coding region. Recently it was reported that 85% of all the transcripts are edited by A-I editing [53], and A-I editing regulated gene expression much more than had been thought.

New A-I editing sites have been found by next-generation sequencing [54]. Also, ADAR1 is now known to frequently target 5′ and 3′ untranslated regions (UTRs) and intronic retrotransposon elements, such as Alu and long interspersed elements (LINE/SINEs). Further, several primary microRNA (miRNA) intermediates undergo A-I editing [55-58]. 99% of the identified A-I editing sites are in non-coding RNA [53]. It was reported that ADARs regulate the expression of microRNA and redirect silencing targets by A-I editing of miRNA [55, 57, 58]. There is extensive interaction between the RNA editing and RNA interference (RNAi) pathways [59]. However, the overview of physiologic significance of non-coding RNA editing still remains to be clarified, including whether those non-coding RNA editing is involved in the pathogenesis of DSH.

Additionally, in these miRNA/siRNA pathways, an editing-independent effect of inhibition of RNAi by ADARs was reported [44].

2.8. DSH murine models

Wang et al. generated an Adar1 knockout (KO) murine model [60] that lacks exons 12–15, corresponding to the catalytic RNA-editing domain. Hartner et al. [61] created a KO mouse that has the homozygous deletion of exons 7-9 or exons 2-13.

In the $Adar^{-/-}$ mouse with homozygous deletion exons 7-9 or exons 2-13, the liver sizes in fatal mice were the same as in wild-type mice until E11.0 - 11.25, and they did not increase further, whereas wild-type and $Adar^{+/-}$ embryo livers enlarged by up to 50% between E11.5 and 12.5 [61]. Reduced cell density and blood accumulation were observed by microscopy in $Adar^{-/-}$ fatal livers, perhaps resulting from massive cell death. Embryonic hematopoietic tissues were significantly reduced in the yolk sac, fetal liver and peripheral blood compared with wild-type and $Adar^{+/-}$ embryos. There were no morphological abnormalities in other tissues [61].

In KO mice with the homozygous deletions of exons 12-15, widespread apoptosis was detected in many tissues of the $Adar^{-/-}$ mouse embryos collected live from E10.5 to E11.5, particularly in the heart, liver and vertebra, despite their normal gross appearance [60]. Fibroblasts derived from $Adar^{-/-}$ embryos were also prone to apoptosis induced by serum deprivation. Those results demonstrated that ADAR1 is essential to embryogenesis and suggested that it functions to promote the survival of numerous tissues by editing one or more double-stranded RNAs required for protection against stress-induced apoptosis [60]].

KO mice with different mutant alleles showed the same result of fatal lethality at E11.5–12.5 [60, 61].

Interestingly nonsense mutations that encode proteins similar to those in the knockout mice have been reported in DSH patients, such as R328X [10] or Y989X [62]. Notably, DSH patients are heterozygous for the *ADAR1* gene mutation that is inherited as a dominant trait. Unlike DSH patients, the $Adar^{+/-}$ mouse, which is heterozygous for Adar1 deletion, does not manifest any clinical abnormalities of the skin, including the face or dorsal sites of the extremities, which are the most noticeable sites of DSH in humans [60, 61]. The effect of ADAR1 gene mutation on skin might be milder in heterozygous mice than in heterozygous humans.

The previously described KO mice had disruptions of both the p110 and p150 isoforms [60, 61]. To circumvent the embryonic lethality associated with simultaneous disruption of p110 and p150, a selective p150-isoform-disrupted mouse was generated in which the promoter and exon 1A region of the p150 isoform of Adar1 were specifically targeted, while the expression of p110 was left intact [63]. Selective disruption of p150 alone resulted in embryonic lethality from E11-E12 [63], similar to the time point of embryonic lethality seen previously with disruption of p110 and p150 [60, 61]. These results indicate that the p150 isoform of ADAR1 plays a critically important role in embryogenesis. Furthermore, they raise the possibility that the embryonic lethality seen in the previously described *Adar1* gene disruptions may have resulted primarily from ablation of p150 expression. This p150-isoform-specific heterozygous KO mouse shows no skin manifestations clinically [63].

To investigate in more depth the role of ADAR1 in skin, an epidermis-specific Adar1 knockout murine model was established [64]. In this model, Adar1 gene deletion was induced by tamoxifen exposure. First we administrated tamoxifen orally to ten K14-Adar1 mice (FVB background) at the age of 6 weeks old for 5 consecutive days. Eight of these treated mice died within three weeks after treatment, developing a phenotype that included dramatically decreased aggressiveness, thin body shape, fur loss, poor skin resiliency, skin rash and bleeding [64]. In the FVB mice, H–E stained sections revealed massive necrosis in the epidermis and few remaining hair follicles in the dermis. Thickening of the interfollicular epidermis (IFE) and the stratum corneum were observed, while skin ulcers were observed in some other areas [64]. In the B6 mice, epidermal necrosis was not observed but increased keratinocytes and thickened stratum corneum were evident. p150-specific Adar1-deleted newborn B6 mouse showed death in a subset of the hair follicles. These results support an essential role for ADAR1 in the epidermis during the first hair follicle developmental cycle [64].

3. Conclusion

The RNA editing mechanism has been gaining much attention. A-I editing has been shown to affect a wide variety of RNA transcripts, both protein coding and noncoding sequences. Its relationship with some neurological diseases, e.g., amyotrophic lateral sclerosis [50, 65-67], epilepsy [68], depression [69] and schizophrenia [70], has been clarified. In the skin, although the expression of ADAR1 is recognized, its function remains unknown. Various functions of ADAR have been successively clarified. In DSH patients, if a new function of ADAR1 or a new target gene of ADAR1 were to be identified, it would not only help to elucidate the pathogenesis of DSH, but also be one step toward clarifying RNA editing in the skin. For dermatologists, it is also very interesting how this characteristic skin manifestation, a mixture of pigmented and depigmented macules with a unique distribution of eruptions in the extremities, develops.

Author details

Michihiro Kono and Masashi Akiyama
Department of Dermatology, Nagoya University Graduate School of Medicine, Nagoya, Japan

4. References

[1] Miyamura Y, Suzuki T, Kono M, Inagaki K, Ito S, Suzuki N, et al. Mutations of the RNA-specific adenosine deaminase gene (DSRAD) are involved in dyschromatosis symmetrica hereditaria. Am J Hum Genet. 2003 Sep;73(3):693-9.
[2] Bass BL, Weintraub H. An unwinding activity that covalently modifies its double-stranded RNA substrate. Cell. 1988 Dec 23;55(6):1089-98.
[3] Wagner RW, Smith JE, Cooperman BS, Nishikura K. A double-stranded RNA unwinding activity introduces structural alterations by means of adenosine to inosine conversions in mammalian cells and Xenopus eggs. Proc Natl Acad Sci U S A. 1989 Apr;86(8):2647-51.
[4] Sommer B, Kohler M, Sprengel R, Seeburg PH. RNA editing in brain controls a determinant of ion flow in glutamate-gated channels. Cell. 1991 Oct 4;67(1):11-9.
[5] Burns CM, Chu H, Rueter SM, Hutchinson LK, Canton H, Sanders-Bush E, et al. Regulation of serotonin-2C receptor G-protein coupling by RNA editing. Nature. 1997 May 15;387(6630):303-8.
[6] Nishikura K. Functions and regulation of RNA editing by ADAR deaminases. Annu Rev Biochem. 2010;79:321-49.

[7] Toyama I. An unknown disorder of hyperpigmentation (in Japanese). Jpn J Dermatol Urol. 1910;10:644.

[8] Toyama I. Dyschromatosis symmetrica hereditaria (in Japanese). Jpn J Dermatol Urol. 1929;29:95–6.

[9] Suzuki N, Suzuki T, Inagaki K, Ito S, Kono M, Fukai K, et al. Mutation analysis of the ADAR1 gene in dyschromatosis symmetrica hereditaria and genetic differentiation from both dyschromatosis universalis hereditaria and acropigmentatio reticularis. J Invest Dermatol. 2005 Jun;124(6):1186-92.

[10] Hou Y, Chen J, Gao M, Zhou F, Du W, Shen Y, et al. Five novel mutations of RNA-specific adenosine deaminase gene with dyschromatosis symmetrica hereditaria. Acta Derm Venereol. 2007;87(1):18-21.

[11] Kantaputra PN, Chinadet W, Ohazama A, Kono M. Dyschromatosis symmetrica hereditaria with long hair on the forearms, hypo/hyperpigmented hair, and dental anomalies: Report of a novel ADAR1 mutation. Am J Med Genet A. 2012 Sep;158A(9):2258-65.

[12] Kim NI, Park SA, Youn JI. Dyschromatosis symmetrica hereditaria affecting two families. Korean J Dermatol. 1980;18:585-9.

[13] Sheu HM, Yu HS. Dyschromatosis symmetrica hereditaria--a histochemical and ultrastructural study. Taiwan Yi Xue Hui Za Zhi. 1985 Feb;84(2):238-49.

[14] Dhar S, Malakar S. Acropigmentation of Dohi in a 12-year-old boy. Pediatr Dermatol. 1998 May-Jun;15(3):242.

[15] Bilen N, Akturk AS, Kawaguchi M, Salman S, Ercin C, Hozumi Y, et al. Dyschromatosis symmetrica hereditaria: A case report from Turkey, a new association and a novel gene mutation. J Dermatol. 2012 Oct;39(10):857-8.

[16] Patrizi A, Manneschi V, Pini A, Baioni E, Ghetti P. Dyschromatosis symmetrica hereditaria associated with idiopathic torsion dystonia. A case report. Acta Derm Venereol. 1994 Mar;74(2):135-7.

[17] Ostlere LS, Ratnavel RC, Lawlor F, Black MM, Griffiths WA. Reticulate acropigmentation of Dohi. Clin Exp Dermatol. 1995 Nov;20(6):477-9.

[18] Kono M, Akiyama M, Suganuma M, Tomita Y. Dyschromatosis symmetrica hereditaria by ADAR1 mutations and viral encephalitis: a hidden link? International Journal of Dermatology. in press.

[19] Tomita Y, Suzuki T. Genetics of pigmentary disorders. Am J Med Genet C Semin Med Genet. 2004 Nov 15;131C(1):75-81.

[20] Oyama M, Shimizu H, Ohata Y, Tajima S, Nishikawa T. Dyschromatosis symmetrica hereditaria (reticulate acropigmentation of Dohi): report of a Japanese family with the condition and a literature review of 185 cases. Br J Dermatol. 1999 Mar;140(3):491-6.

[21] Kondo T, Suzuki T, Ito S, Kono M, Negoro T, Tomita Y. Dyschromatosis symmetrica hereditaria associated with neurological disorders. J Dermatol. 2008 Oct;35(10):662-6.

[22] Liu Q, Jiang L, Liu WL, Kang XJ, Ao Y, Sun M, et al. Two novel mutations and evidence for haploinsufficiency of the ADAR gene in dyschromatosis symmetrica hereditaria. Br J Dermatol. 2006 Apr;154(4):636-42.

[23] Kondo T, Suzuki T, Mitsuhashi Y, Ito S, Kono M, Komine M, et al. Six novel mutations of the ADAR1 gene in patients with dyschromatosis symmetrica hereditaria: histological observation and comparison of genotypes and clinical phenotypes. J Dermatol. 2008 Jul;35(7):395-406.
[24] Nishigori C, Miyachi Y, Takebe H, Imamura S. A case of xeroderma pigmentosum with clinical appearance of dyschromatosis symmetrica hereditaria. Pediatr Dermatol. 1986 Nov;3(5):410-3.
[25] Satoh Y, Yoshida M. Clinical and photobiological differences between dyschromatosis symmetrica hereditaria and xeroderma pigmentosum. J Dermatol. 1980 Oct;7(5):317-22.
[26] Hata S, Yokomi I. Density of dopa-positive melanocytes in dyschromatosis symmetrica hereditaria. Dermatologica. 1985;171(1):27-9.
[27] Melcher T, Maas S, Herb A, Sprengel R, Seeburg PH, Higuchi M. A mammalian RNA editing enzyme. Nature. 1996 Feb 1;379(6564):460-4.
[28] Chen CX, Cho DS, Wang Q, Lai F, Carter KC, Nishikura K. A third member of the RNA-specific adenosine deaminase gene family, ADAR3, contains both single- and double-stranded RNA binding domains. Rna. 2000 May;6(5):755-67.
[29] Kim U, Wang Y, Sanford T, Zeng Y, Nishikura K. Molecular cloning of cDNA for double-stranded RNA adenosine deaminase, a candidate enzyme for nuclear RNA editing. Proc Natl Acad Sci U S A. 1994 Nov 22;91(24):11457-61.
[30] Patterson JB, Samuel CE. Expression and regulation by interferon of a double-stranded-RNA-specific adenosine deaminase from human cells: evidence for two forms of the deaminase. Mol Cell Biol. 1995 Oct;15(10):5376-88.
[31] Patterson JB, Thomis DC, Hans SL, Samuel CE. Mechanism of interferon action: double-stranded RNA-specific adenosine deaminase from human cells is inducible by alpha and gamma interferons. Virology. 1995 Jul 10;210(2):508-11.
[32] Rueter SM, Dawson TR, Emeson RB. Regulation of alternative splicing by RNA editing. Nature. 1999 May 6;399(6731):75-80.
[33] Higuchi M, Single FN, Kohler M, Sommer B, Sprengel R, Seeburg PH. RNA editing of AMPA receptor subunit GluR-B: a base-paired intron-exon structure determines position and efficiency. Cell. 1993 Dec 31;75(7):1361-70.
[34] Lomeli H, Mosbacher J, Melcher T, Hoger T, Geiger JR, Kuner T, et al. Control of kinetic properties of AMPA receptor channels by nuclear RNA editing. Science. 1994 Dec 9;266(5191):1709-13.
[35] Polson AG, Bass BL, Casey JL. RNA editing of hepatitis delta virus antigenome by dsRNA-adenosine deaminase. Nature. 1996 Apr 4;380(6573):454-6.
[36] Li JB, Levanon EY, Yoon JK, Aach J, Xie B, Leproust E, et al. Genome-wide identification of human RNA editing sites by parallel DNA capturing and sequencing. Science. 2009 May 29;324(5931):1210-3.
[37] Kono M, Akiyama M, Kondo T, Suzuki T, Suganuma M, Wataya-Kaneda M, et al. Four novel ADAR1 gene mutations in patients with dyschromatosis symmetrica hereditaria. J Dermatol. 2012;39(9):819-21.

[38] Lai F, Drakas R, Nishikura K. Mutagenic analysis of double-stranded RNA adenosine deaminase, a candidate enzyme for RNA editing of glutamate-gated ion channel transcripts. J Biol Chem. 1995 Jul 21;270(29):17098-105.

[39] Suzuki N, Suzuki T, Inagaki K, Ito S, Kono M, Horikawa T, et al. Ten novel mutations of the ADAR1 gene in Japanese patients with dyschromatosis symmetrica hereditaria. J Invest Dermatol. 2007 Feb;127(2):309-11.

[40] Cho DS, Yang W, Lee JT, Shiekhattar R, Murray JM, Nishikura K. Requirement of dimerization for RNA editing activity of adenosine deaminases acting on RNA. J Biol Chem. 2003 May 9;278(19):17093-102.

[41] Valente L, Nishikura K. RNA binding-independent dimerization of adenosine deaminases acting on RNA and dominant negative effects of nonfunctional subunits on dimer functions. J Biol Chem. 2007 Jun 1;282(22):16054-61.

[42] Tojo K, Sekijima Y, Suzuki T, Suzuki N, Tomita Y, Yoshida K, et al. Dystonia, mental deterioration, and dyschromatosis symmetrica hereditaria in a family with ADAR1 mutation. Mov Disord. 2006 Sep;21(9):1510-3.

[43] Macbeth MR, Schubert HL, Vandemark AP, Lingam AT, Hill CP, Bass BL. Inositol hexakisphosphate is bound in the ADAR2 core and required for RNA editing. Science. 2005 Sep 2;309(5740):1534-9.

[44] Heale BS, Keegan LP, McGurk L, Michlewski G, Brindle J, Stanton CM, et al. Editing independent effects of ADARs on the miRNA/siRNA pathways. Embo J. 2009 Oct 21;28(20):3145-56.

[45] Heale BS, Keegan LP, O'Connell MA. ADARs have effects beyond RNA editing. Cell Cycle. 2009 Dec 15;8(24):4011-2.

[46] Bischoff S, Barhanin J, Bettler B, Mulle C, Heinemann S. Spatial distribution of kainate receptor subunit mRNA in the mouse basal ganglia and ventral mesencephalon. J Comp Neurol. 1997 Mar 24;379(4):541-62.

[47] Nobrega JN, Raymond R, Barlow K, Hamann M, Richter A. Changes in AMPA receptor binding in an animal model of inborn paroxysmal dystonia. Exp Neurol. 2002 Aug;176(2):371-6.

[48] Richter A, Loscher W, Loschmann PA. The AMPA receptor antagonist NBQX exerts antidystonic effects in an animal model of idiopathic dystonia. Eur J Pharmacol. 1993 Feb 9;231(2):287-91.

[49] Wang Q, Khillan J, Gadue P, Nishikura K. Requirement of the RNA editing deaminase ADAR1 gene for embryonic erythropoiesis. Science. 2000 Dec 1;290(5497):1765-8.

[50] Kwak S, Kawahara Y. Deficient RNA editing of GluR2 and neuronal death in amyotropic lateral sclerosis. J Mol Med (Berl). 2005 Feb;83(2):110-20.

[51] Kim KM, Herrera GA, Battarbee HD. Role of glutaraldehyde in calcification of porcine aortic valve fibroblasts. Am J Pathol. 1999 Mar;154(3):843-52.

[52] Manyam BV, Walters AS, Narla KR. Bilateral striopallidodentate calcinosis: clinical characteristics of patients seen in a registry. Mov Disord. 2001 Mar;16(2):258-64.

[53] Athanasiadis A, Rich A, Maas S. Widespread A-to-I RNA editing of Alu-containing mRNAs in the human transcriptome. PLoS Biol. 2004 Dec;2(12):e391.

[54] Eggington JM, Greene T, Bass BL. Predicting sites of ADAR editing in double-stranded RNA. Nat Commun. 2011;2:319.

[55] Yang W, Chendrimada TP, Wang Q, Higuchi M, Seeburg PH, Shiekhattar R, et al. Modulation of microRNA processing and expression through RNA editing by ADAR deaminases. Nat Struct Mol Biol. 2006 Jan;13(1):13-21.

[56] Kawahara Y, Nishikura K. Extensive adenosine-to-inosine editing detected in Alu repeats of antisense RNAs reveals scarcity of sense-antisense duplex formation. FEBS Lett. 2006 Apr 17;580(9):2301-5.

[57] Kawahara Y, Zinshteyn B, Sethupathy P, Iizasa H, Hatzigeorgiou AG, Nishikura K. Redirection of silencing targets by adenosine-to-inosine editing of miRNAs. Science. 2007 Feb 23;315(5815):1137-40.

[58] Kawahara Y, Zinshteyn B, Chendrimada TP, Shiekhattar R, Nishikura K. RNA editing of the microRNA-151 precursor blocks cleavage by the Dicer-TRBP complex. EMBO Rep. 2007 Aug;8(8):763-9.

[59] Nishikura K. Editor meets silencer: crosstalk between RNA editing and RNA interference. Nat Rev Mol Cell Biol. 2006 Dec;7(12):919-31.

[60] Wang Q, Miyakoda M, Yang W, Khillan J, Stachura DL, Weiss MJ, et al. Stress-induced apoptosis associated with null mutation of ADAR1 RNA editing deaminase gene. J Biol Chem. 2004 Feb 6;279(6):4952-61.

[61] Hartner JC, Schmittwolf C, Kispert A, Muller AM, Higuchi M, Seeburg PH. Liver disintegration in the mouse embryo caused by deficiency in the RNA-editing enzyme ADAR1. J Biol Chem. 2004 Feb 6;279(6):4894-902.

[62] Murata I, Hozumi Y, Kawaguchi M, Katagiri Y, Yasumoto S, Kubo Y, et al. Four novel mutations of the ADAR1 gene in dyschromatosis symmetrica hereditaria. J Dermatol Sci. 2009 Jan;53(1):76-7.

[63] Ward SV, George CX, Welch MJ, Liou LY, Hahm B, Lewicki H, et al. RNA editing enzyme adenosine deaminase is a restriction factor for controlling measles virus replication that also is required for embryogenesis. Proc Natl Acad Sci U S A. 2011 Jan 4;108(1):331-6.

[64] Sharma R, Wang Y, Zhou P, Steinman RA, Wang Q. An essential role of RNA editing enzyme ADAR1 in mouse skin. J Dermatol Sci. 2011 Oct;64(1):70-2.

[65] Kawahara Y, Kwak S, Sun H, Ito K, Hashida H, Aizawa H, et al. Human spinal motoneurons express low relative abundance of GluR2 mRNA: an implication for excitotoxicity in ALS. J Neurochem. 2003 May;85(3):680-9.

[66] Kawahara Y, Ito K, Sun H, Aizawa H, Kanazawa I, Kwak S. Glutamate receptors: RNA editing and death of motor neurons. Nature. 2004 Feb 26;427(6977):801.

[67] Kawahara Y, Kwak S. Excitotoxicity and ALS: what is unique about the AMPA receptors expressed on spinal motor neurons? Amyotroph Lateral Scler Other Motor Neuron Disord. 2005 Sep;6(3):131-44.

[68] Delorenzo RJ, Sun DA, Deshpande LS. Cellular mechanisms underlying acquired epilepsy: the calcium hypothesis of the induction and maintainance of epilepsy. Pharmacol Ther. 2005 Mar;105(3):229-66.

[69] Iwamoto K, Nakatani N, Bundo M, Yoshikawa T, Kato T. Altered RNA editing of serotonin 2C receptor in a rat model of depression. Neurosci Res. 2005 Sep;53(1):69-76.

[70] Dracheva S, Elhakem SL, Marcus SM, Siever LJ, McGurk SR, Haroutunian V. RNA editing and alternative splicing of human serotonin 2C receptor in schizophrenia. J Neurochem. 2003 Dec;87(6):1402-12.

Chapter 10

Genetics of Epidermodysplasia Verruciformis

Masaaki Kawase

Additional information is available at the end of the chapter

http://dx.doi.org/10.5772/55340

1. Introduction

Epidermodysplasia verruciformis (EV; MIM#226400) is a genodermatosis characterized by susceptibility to epidermodysplasia verruciformis-human papillomavirus (EV-HPV) infections which leads to early development of disseminated pityriasis versicolor-like and flat wart-like lesions [1]. The disease was first described by Lewandowski and Lutz in [1]. Approximately half of all patients with EV will develop cutaneous malignancies, predominately Bowen's type carcinoma in situ and invasive squamous cell carcinomas that occur mainly on sun-exposed areas in the fourth or fifth decade of life [2-4].Thus, EV is in essence a genetic cancer of viral origin, and could also be regarded as a model of cutaneous HPV oncogenesis [5, 6]. In general, EV shows an autosomal recessive pattern of inheritance [7]. The EV loci were mapped to chromosome 2p21-p24 (EV2) and 17q25 (EV1) [8], respectively. In the EV1 interval, 2 adjacent related genes, EVER1 and EVER2, were identified in 2002 [9]. EVER proteins are members of transmembrane channel-like (TMC) family. They are encoded by 8 genes (TMC1-8). EVER1 and EVER2 correspond to TMC6 and TMC8, respectively [10, 11]. Therefore the recent literature has focused on the mutation finding the culpable gene. Clinical and histologic findings, EV-HPV, cutaneous oncogenesis, and genetics will be briefly reviewed.

2. Clinical and histologic findings

Classic EV begins during childhood with highly polymorphic cutaneous lesions, including pityriasis versicolor-like macules (Figure 1), flat wart-like papules (Figure 2), and lesions resembling seborrheic keratoses that can undergo malignant transformation [2, 4, 6, 12, 13]. Approximately half of all patients with EV will develop cutaneous malignancies, predominately Bowen's type carcinoma in situ and invasive squamous cell carcinomas (SCCs) that occur mainly on sun-exposed areas in the fourth or fifth decade of life [2, 4, 6, 12]. Development of malignant transformation is usually associated with HPV-5 and -8.

However, the mechanism of carcinogenesis induced by EV-related HPV types is not clear in contrast to the other oncogenic HPVs, these do not seem to need integration into the host's genome [14]. EV patients have impaired cell-mediated immunity (CMI) [15–20]. Decreased T-lymphocyte counts and CD4/CD8 ratios and a reduced T-cell responsiveness to mitogens were found in some patients.

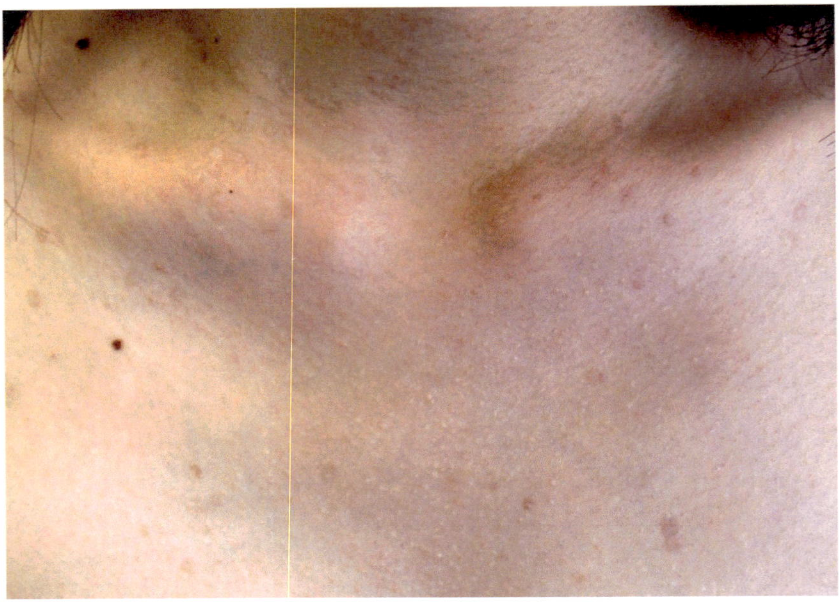

Figure 1. Pityriasis versicolor-like macules

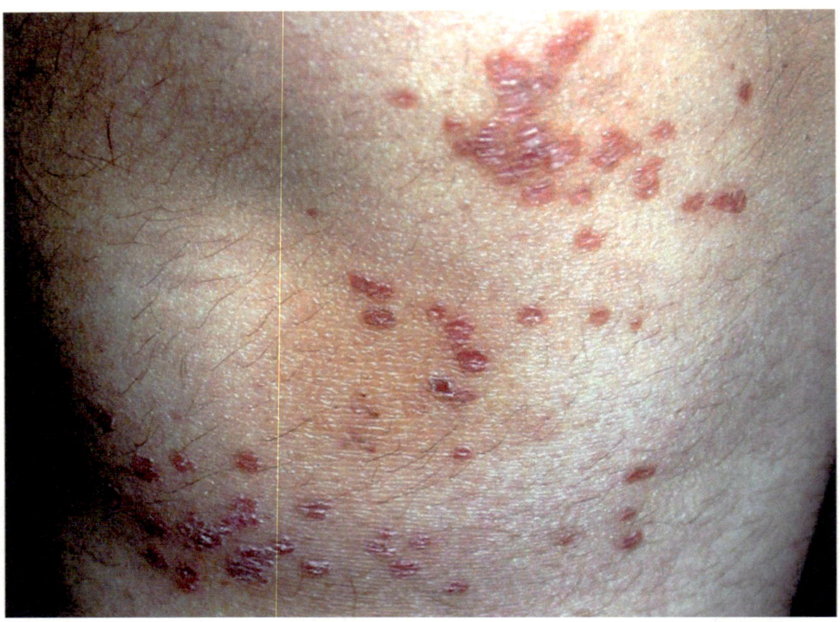

Figure 2. Flat wart-like papules

There is an indication of EV-like disease being a result of exogenous immunodeficiency in HIV infection and in the patients with immunodeficiency states(e.g. following renal transplantation, in systemic lupus erythematosus or Hodgkin's disease) [21-24].This form has been named "acquired epidermodysplasia verruciformis" [25].

Histopathologically, lesions demonstrate stereotypical enlarged keratinocytes in upper epidermis with gray-blue cytoplasm, enlarged round nuclei with pale chromatin, and one or multiple nucleoli (Figure 3).The Immunohistochemistry findings showed the HPV antigens

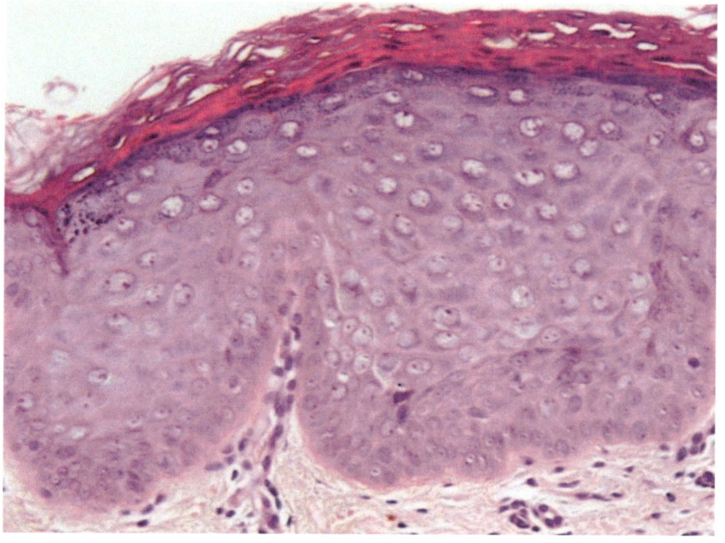

Figure 3. Enlarged keratinocytes in upper epidermis with gray-blue cytoplasm (haematoxylin and eosin)

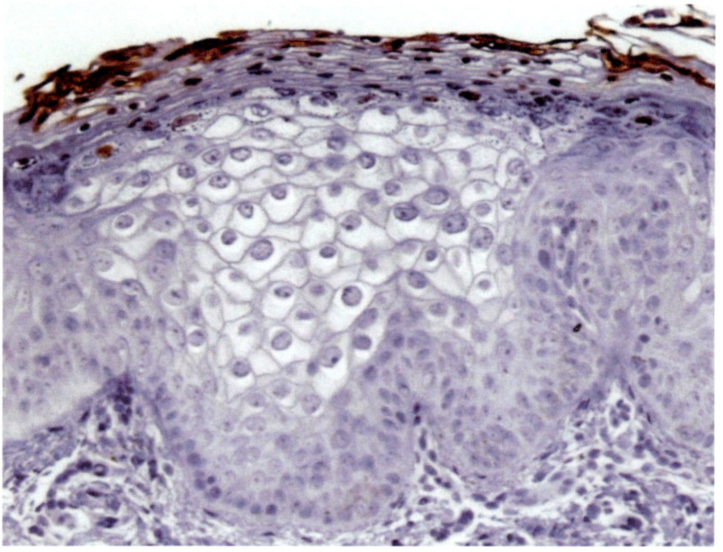

Figure 4. HPV antigens using anti-HPV monoclonal antibody are demonstrated

using anti-HPV monoclonal antibody (K1H8) were located in the cell nucleus of the third superior of the epithelium, observing the brownish-gold colored precipitins caused by cromogen in the nucleus of these cells (Figure 4). In *in situ* hybridization (ISH) EV HPV-5 DNA was detected in upper epidermis, abundant in parakeratotic cells (Figure 5) [26].In electron microscopy, The nuclei are clarified with maeginated chromatin, and crystalline viral particles are present in nucleoplasm and in the prominent nucleoli (Figure 6). Under an electron microscope, HPV5 virions purified from pooled scales of EV patients and virus-like particles (VLP) assembled from a purified recombinant baculoviruses expressing the L1 major capsid protein of HPV5 were observed(Figure 7) [27].

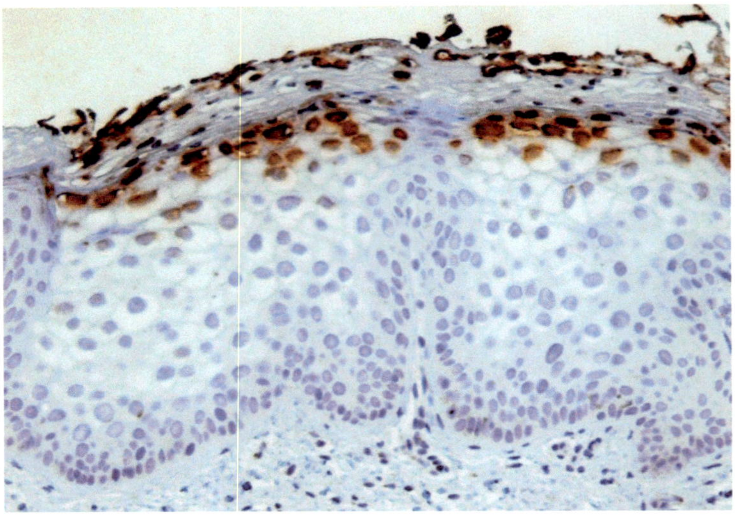

Figure 5. HPV-5 DNA is demonstrated in the nuclei of spinous and granular cells (ISH)

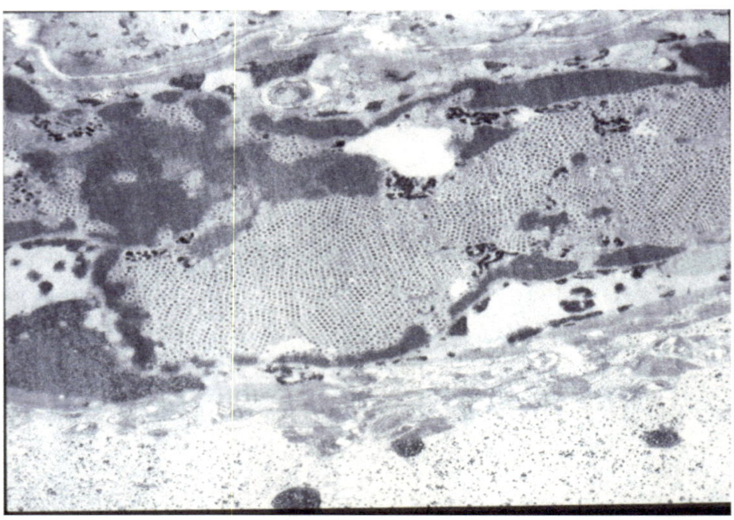

Figure 6. Crystalline viral particles in electron microscopy

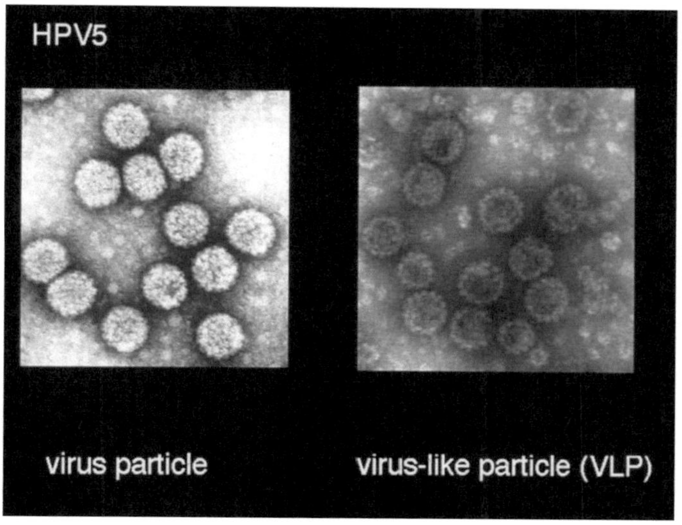

Figure 7.

3. EV-HPV infection

The disease is a generalized HPV infection, resulting from a genetically determined susceptibility of the skin to infection with particular types of HPV [28]. Papillomaviruses (PVs) are small, non-enveloped, double-stranded DNA viruses, which can infect mucosal or cutaneous epithelia. At least 118 distinct papillomavirus (PVs) types, more than 100 of them isolated from humans, have been completely described. The human papillomavirus genotypes are distributed across 5 genera. The five genera encompassing human PV are called alpha (both mucosal and cutaneous types), beta, gamma, mu and nu (exclusively cutaneous types)[29]. Genera are divided into species and types on the basis of nucleotidic sequence comparisons. Members of species have similar biological or pathological properties (Table 1) [29-31]. EV HPV genotypes constitute the beta-papillomavirus genus and are distributed into five species [29, 31], mainly beta 1, comprising the potentially oncogenic types 5, 8, 14, 20, and 47 [2], and beta 2(Table 1). Beta PV are ubiquitous in the general population and frequently establish themselves already during the first weeks of life. Hair follicles are regarded as natural reservoir. About 25% of beta PV detected in adults persist for at least 9 months. Due to very low virus production, seroconversion against beta PV starts sluggishly. Hyperproliferation of keratinocytes in psoriasis patients or after severe burn stimulates virus replication. Massive virus replication only occurs in EV patients, associated with the induction of disseminated skin lesions with a high risk of malignant conversion.

Papillomaviruses share the same genetic organization [32]. At least eight open reading frames (ORFs) are located on the same DNA strand, downstream of a noncoding, long regulatory region containing transcriptional and replication regulatory elements. The E1 and E2 ORFs encode proteins involved in the replication of the viral genome (E1, E2), the segregation of the viral genome in dividing cells (E2) and in the regulation of its transcription (E2). The E6 and E7 proteins interact with cell cycle regulatory proteins and are required for promoting the S-phase and for inhibiting apoptosis in resting and in terminally differentiating keratinocytes. The E6 and E7 proteins of potentially oncogenic genotypes induce genetic and chromosomal instability. The E5 protein displays growth promoting properties. The L1 and L2 ORFs encode the major (L1) and minor (L2) capsid proteins [32]. The genomes of EV HPVs are characterized by a shorter size and a specific organization of the regulatory region, the lack of an E5 ORF [33], and a great intratype genetic heterogeneity [34, 35].

Genus	Spiecies	Human papillomavirus(HPV)
β-papillomavirus	β- 1	**HPV-5,** -8, -14,-12, -19, -20, -21, -24, -25, -36, -47, -93, -98, -99, -105, -118, -124
	β- 2	**HPV-9,** -15, -17, -22, -23, -37, -38, -80, -100, -104, -107, -110, -111, -113, -120, -122, -151
	β- 3	**HPV-49**, -75, -76, -115
	β- 4	**HPV-92**
	β- 5	**HPV-96,** -150

Table 1. HPV-Type in 5 species of the genusβ-Papillomavirus

4. Cutaneous oncogenesis –EV and non-EV

Highly sensitive PCR methods based on various sets of primers have been designed to detect a broad range of known EV HPVs or putative novel EV HPV-related genotypes [36]. This has brought a wealth of information about the epidemiology and biology of these viruses [37, 38]. EV HPVs were found to be highly prevalent in the normal skin of healthy adults [39–41] and shown to be acquired very early in infancy [42]. An impressive diversity of putative novel beta PV has been disclosed [41].

Nonmelanoma skin cancer (NMSC) is the most common form of malignancy in fair-skinned populations. The role of ultraviolet radiation as an environmental carcinogen, capable of inducing mutations in both genomic and mitochondrial DNA and thereby being a causative agent in the development of NMSC, is well established [43]. Although the importance of HPV in cervical SCC is well-documented, the role of HPV in cutaneous SCC is controversial [43, 44]. EV may offer a model for cutaneous SCC [28]. In both their benign and malignant lesions, a broad spectrum of predominantly beta PV were found with a combined prevalence of 90% for HPV 5 and 8 in SCC [2, 6] . In lesions of EV patients, the viral genome usually persists extrachromosomally and in high copy numbers (100–300 copies per cell equivalent) [45-47]. High viral loads have also been found in hair bulbs from plucked eyebrows of these patients [47]. In both immunocompetent and immunosuppressed non-EV patients these viruses are also frequently found; however, only very low copy numbers (usually below one copy per cell) were detected in actinic keratosis, SCC, basal cell carcinoma, and perilesional skin [48]. It has been shown that beta PV are transcriptionally active in benign and malignant lesions of EV patients [49, 50] and also in 3 of 4 actinic keratosis and 5 of 18 SCC of immunosuppressed non-EV patients [51, 52].

5. Genetics

As early as 1933, Cockayne postulated that EV was probably transmitted by a recessive gene [53] and an autosomal recessive mode of transmission was first proposed in 1972 [54].

Inspections of EV patient pedigrees have revealed that a large portion (approximately 10% in a review of 147 case reports [7]) are born to consanguineous parents. Additionally, because the proportion of EV siblings in families has approached 30% [55], the mode of EV transmission has been thought to be autosomal recessive. An X-linked recessive inheritance has also been reported [56], however, pointing to a possible genetic heterogeneity of the disease [57]. Recent studies have advanced our understanding of the genetic defects carried by EV patients. A genome-wide linkage study was performed recently on consanguineous EV families (first-cousin marriages), using the homozygosity mapping approach that represents a simple and efficient strategy to map rare human recessive traits [8, 58].The two susceptibility loci EV1 and EV2 were first mapped to chromosomes 17q25 from the study of families from Algeria and Colombia and 2p21-p24 from French family, respectively, in 2000 [8]. Since those initial findings were reported, specific mutations in the genes EVER1 and EVER2, both located within the EV1 locus, have been discovered. Ramoz et al. [9] first described two highly conserved nonsense mutations in the EVER1 and EVER2 genes of all affected individuals in two Algerian and two Colombian consanguineous families. Subsequently, novel mutations in these genes were identified in patients of multiple races and nationalities [59-68,9]. In all, 15 truncating, loss-of-function mutations caused by several mechanisms (nonsense mutation, single nucleotide deletion, splice site mutation, and exon deletion) have been identified, eight in EVER1 and seven in EVER2. The *TMC* (transmembrane channel-like) gene family comprises eight genes (TMC1 to8) [10, 11]. EVER1 and EVER2 are identical to the TMC6 and TMC8 genes, respectively. Although the proteins encoded by the EVER genes have been shown to localize in the endoplasmic reticulum with features of integral membrane proteins, the exact function in development of persistent HPV infections has not yet been revealed [9,59]. It has been hypothesized that these proteins act as restriction factors for EV specific HPVs in keratinocytes, and that EV represents a primary deficiency of intrinsic immunity against certain papillomaviruses[57]. Although most EV patients studied (75.6%, according to collaborative efforts reported in the review by [57]) have been found to have homozygous mutations in EVER1 or EVER2, this still leaves a significant number of EV patients with unexplained inheritance patterns. Three cases have reported genetic analysis of EV patients in whom EVER1 or EVER2 mutations were lacking [69-71]. In a recent case-control study, EVER2 polymorphisms were associated with SCC development [66]. The exact function of TMC proteins still unclear, but it is assumed that they belong to a new group of channels or iron transporters and could be involved in signal transduction [10, 11]. EVER1/TMC6 and EVER2/TMC8 proteins are located in the endoplasmic reticulum of keratinocytes, where they form a complex with zinc transporter-1 (ZnT-1). EVER1/TMC6 and EVER2/TMC8 act as modifiers of zinc transporter ZnT-1. Potentially, EVER proteins mediate the protection against oncogenic HPV via regulation of cellular zinc balance [72, 73]. A mutation in the EVER1 or EVER2 gene might block the formation of the EVER/ZnT-1 complex, which would allow the expression of transcription factors (e.g.AP-1), thus promoting viral replication [14].

6. Conclusion

In EV patients there is a strong association between beta HPV infection and NMSC. This predisposition is genetically determined by mutations of the 2 genes EVER1/TMC6 and EVER2/TMC8. However, only in 75% of EV patients, an EVER mutation has been found. This suggests other genes are involved. A second EV susceptibility locus (EV2) on chromosome 2p21-p24 by autosomal recessive inheritance is assumed [8]. X-linked recessive inheritance [56] and autosomal dominant transmission have been reported [71]. Identification of additional genes associated with EV should provide more clues for the understanding of host defences against papillomaviruses.

Author details

Masaaki Kawase
Department of Dermatology, The Jikei University School of Medicine
Nishi-shimbashi, Minato-ku Tokyo, Japan

7. References

[1] Lewandowsky F, Lutz W. Ein Fall einer bisher nicht beschriebenen Hauterkrankung (Epidermodysplasia verruciformis). Arch Dermatol Syphilol 1922; 141 193-203.
[2] Orth G. Epidermodysplasia verruciformis. In: Howley PM, Salzman NP, (ed.) The papovaviridae, vol 2. The papillomaviruses. New York: Plenum Press Inc.; 1987. p199-243.
[3] Orth G, Jablonska S, Favre M, Croissant O, Jarzabek-Chorzelska M, Rzesa G. Characterization of two types of human papillomaviruses in lesions of epidermodysplasia verruciformis. Proc Natl Acad Sci USA 1978; 75 1537-41.
[4] Majewski S, Jablonska S, Orth G. Epidermodysplasia verruciformis. Immunological and nonimmunological surveillance mechanisms: role in tumor progression. Clin Dermatol 1997; 15 321-334.
[5] Jablonska S, Dabrowski J, Jakubowicz K. Epidermodysplasia verruciformis as a model in studies on the role of papovaviruses in oncogenesis. Cancer Res 1972; 32 583-589.
[6] Majewski S, Jablonska S. Epidermodysplasia verruciformis as a model of human papillomavirus-induced genetic cancer of the skin. Arch Dermatol 1995; 131 1312-1318.
[7] Lutzner MA. Epidermodysplasia verruciformis: An autosomal recessive disease characterized by viral warts and skin cancer. A model for viral oncogenesis. Bull Cancer 1978; 65 169-182.
[8] Ramoz N, Taïeb A, Rueda LA, Montoya LS, Bouadjar B, Favre M, Orth G. Evidence for a nonallelic heterogeneity of epidermodysplasia verruciformis with two susceptibility loci mapped to chromosome regions 2p21-p24 and 17q25. J Invest Dermatol 2000; 114 1148-1153.
[9] Ramoz N, Rueda LA, Bouadjar B, Montoya LS, Orth G, Favre M. Mutations in two adjacent novel genes are associated with epidermodysplasia verruciformis. Nat Genet 2002; 32 579-581.
[10] Kurima K, Yang Y, Sorber K, Griffith AJ. Characterization of the transmembrane channel-like (*TMC*) gene family: functional clues from hearing loss and epidermodysplasia verruciformis. Genomics 2003; 82 300-308.

[11] Keresztes G, Mutai H, Heller S. *TMC* and *EVER* genes belong to a larger novel family, the TMC gene family encoding transmembrane proteins. BMC Genomics 2003; 4 24-35.
[12] Cockayne EA. Inherited abnormalities of the skin and its appendages.London: Oxford University Press; 1933. p156.
[13] Jacyk WK, Dreyer L, de Villiers EM. Seborrheic Keratoses of Black Patients with Epidermodysplasia Verruciformis Contain Human papillomavirus DNA. Am J Dermatopathol 1993; 15(1) 1-6.
[14] Lazarczyk M, Cassonnet P, Pons C, Jacob Y, Favre M. EVER proteins as a natural barrier against papillomaviruses: a new insight into the pathogenesis of human papillomavirus infections. Microbiol Mol Biol Rev 2009; 73(2) 348-370.
[15] GlinskiW, Jablonska S, Langner A, Obalek S, Haftek M, Proniewska M. Cell-mediated immunity in epidermodysplasia verruciformis. Dermatologica 1976; 153 218-227.
[16] Prawer SE, Pass F, Vance JC, Greenberg LJ, Yunis EJ, Zelickson AS. Depressed immune function in epidermodysplasia verruciformis. Arch Dermatol 1977; 113 495-499.
[17] Oliveira WRP, Carrasco S, Neto CF, Rady P, Tyring SK. Nonspecific cellmediated immunity in patients with epidermodysplasia verruciformis. J Dermatol 2003; 30 203-209.
[18] Glinski W, Obalek S, Jablonska S, Orth G. T-cell defect in patients with epidermodysplasia verruciformis due to human papillomavirus types 3 and 5. Dermatologica 1981; 162 141-147.
[19] Majewski S, Skopinska-Rozewska E, Jabłonska S, Wasik M, Misiewicz J, Orth G. Partial defects of cell-mediated immunity in patients with epidermodysplasia verruciformis. J Am Acad Dermatol 1986; 15 966–973.
[20] Majewski S, Jablonska S. Epidermodysplasia verruciformis as a model of human papillomavirus-induced genetic cancers: The role of local immunosurveillance. Am J Med Sci 1992; 304 174-179.
[21] Berger TG, Sawchuk WS, Leonardi C, Langenberg A, Tappero J, Leboit PE. Epidermodysplasia verruciformis-associated papillomavirus infection complicating human immunodeficiency virus disease. Br J Dermatol 1991; 124(1) 79-83.
[22] Barr BB, Benton EC, McLaren K, Bunney MH, Smith IW, Blessing K, Hunter JA. Human papillomavirus infection and skin cancer in renal allograft recipients. Lancet 1989; 21(1) 124-129.
[23] Gross G, Ellinger K, Roussaki A, Fuchs PG, Peter HH, Pfister H. Epidermodysplasia verruciformis in a patient with Hodgkin's disease: characterization of a new papillomavirus type and interferon treatment.J Invest Dermatol 1988; 91(1) 43-48.
[24] Tanigaki T, Kanda R, Sato K. Epidermodysplasia verruciformis (L-L, 1922) in a patient with systemic lupus erythematosus. Arch Dermatol Res 1986; 278(3) 247-248.
[25] Rogers HD, Macgregor JL, Nord KM, Tyring S, Rady P, Engler DE, Grossman ME. Acquired epidermodysplasia verruciformis. J Am Acad Dermatol 2009; 60(2) 315-320.
[26] Kawase M, Honda M, Niimura M. Detection of human papillomavirus type 60 in plantar cysts and verruca plantaris by the in situ hybridization method using digoxigenin labeled probes. J Dermatol 1994; 21(10) 709-715.
[27] Kawase M. Self-assembly of the major capsid L1 protein of human papillomavirus type 5 into virus-like particles in insect cells. Tokyo Jikeikai Medical Journal 1996; 111 75-83.
[28] Majewski S, Jabłońska S. Epidermodysplasia verruciformis as a model of human papillomavirus-induced genetic cancer of the skin. Arch Dermatol 1995; 131(11) 1312-1318.

[29] de Villiers EM, Fauquet C, Broker TR, Bernard HU, zur Hausen H. Classification of papillomaviruses. Virology 2004; 324 17-27.

[30] Schiffman M, Herrero R, Desalle R, Hildesheim A, Wacholder S, Rodriguez AC, Bratti MC, Sherman ME, Morales J, Guillen D, Alfaro M, Hutchinson M, Wright TC, Solomon D, Chen Z, Schussler J, Castle PE, Burk RD. The carcinogenicity of human papillomavirus types reflects viral evolution. Virology 2005; 337 76-84.

[31] Bernard HU, Burk RD, Chen Z, van Doorslaer K, Hausen Hz, de Villiers EM. Classification of papillomaviruses (PVs) based on 189 PV types and proposal of taxonomic amendments. Virology 2010; 401(1) 70-79.

[32] Howley PM, Lowy DR. Papillomaviruses and their replication. In: Knipe DM, Howley PM, Griffin DE, Lamb RA, Martin MA, Roizman B, Straus SE., (ed.) Fields Virology. 4th ed. Philadelphia: Lippincott Williams &Wilkins; 2001. p2197-2330.

[33] Fuchs PG, Pfister H. Papillomaviruses in epidermodysplasia verruciformis. In: Lacey C, (ed.) Papillomavirus reviews: Current research on papillomaviruses. Leeds: Leeds University Press; 1996. p253-261.

[34] Deau MC, Favre M, Orth G. Genetic heterogeneity among human papillomaviruses (HPV) associated with epidermodysplasia verruciformis: evidence for multiple allelic forms of HPV5 and HPV8 E6 genes. Virology 1991; 184 492-503.

[35] Kawase M, Orth G, Jablonska S, Blanchet-Bardon C, Rueda LA, Favre M. Variability and phylogeny of the L1 capsid protein gene of human papillomavirus type 5: contribution of clusters of nonsynonymous mutations and of a 30-nucleotide duplication. Virology 1996; 221(1) 189-198.

[36] de Koning M, Quint W, Struijk L, Kleter B, Wanningen P, van Doorn LJ, Weissenborn SJ, Feltkamp M, ter Schegget J. Evaluation of a novel highly sensitive, broad-spectrum PCR-reverse hybridization assay for detection and identification of beta-papillomavirus DNA. J Clin Microbiol 2006; 44 1792-1800.

[37] Orth G. Human papillomaviruses and the skin: More to be learned. J Invest Dermatol 2004; 123:XI-III.

[38] Orth G. Human papillomaviruses associated with epidermodysplasia verruciformis in nonmelanoma skin cancers: Guilty or innocent? J Invest Dermatol 2005; 125:XII-II.

[39] Boxman IL, Berkhout RJ, Mulder LH, Wolkers MC, Bouwes Bavinck JN, Vermeer BJ, ter Schegget J. Detection of human papillomavirusDNA in plucked hairs from renal transplant recipients and healthy volunteers. J Invest Dermatol 1997; 108 712-715.

[40] Astori G, Lavergne D, Benton C, Höckmayr B, Egawa K, Garbe C, de Villiers EM. Human papillomaviruses are commonly found in normal skin of immunocompetent hosts. J Invest Dermatol 1998; 110 752–755.

[41] Antonsson A, Forslund O, Ekberg H, Sterner G, Hansson BG. The ubiquity and impressive genomic diversity of human skin papillomaviruses suggest a commensalic nature of these viruses. J Virol 2000; 74 11636-11641.

[42] Antonsson A, Karanfilovska S, Lindqvist PG, Hansson BG. General acquisition of human papillomavirus infections of skin occurs in early infancy. J Clin Microbiol 2003; 41 2509-2514.

[43] Akgul B, Cooke JC, Storey A. HPV-associated skin disease. J Pathol 2006; 208 165-175.

[44] Gewirtzman A, Bartlett B, Tyring S. Epidermodysplasia verruciformis and human papilloma virus. Curr Opin Infect Dis 2008; 21 141-146.

[45] Pfister H. Chapter 8: Human papillomavirus and skin cancer. J Natl Cancer Inst Monogr 2003; 31 52-56.

[46] Orth G. Genetics of epidermodysplasia verruciformis: insights into host defense against papillomaviruses. Semin Immunol 2006; 18 362-374.

[47] Dell'Oste V, Azzimonti B, De Andrea M, Mondini M, Zavattaro E, Leigheb G, Weissenborn SJ, Pfister H, Michael KM, Waterboer T, Pawlita M, Amantea A, Landolfo S, Gariglio M. High beta-HPV DNA loads and strong seroreactivity are present in epidermodysplasia verruciformis. J Invest Dermatol 2009; 129:1026-1034.

[48] Weissenborn SJ, Nindl I, Purdie K, Harwood C, Proby C, Breuer J, Majewski S, Pfister H, Wieland U. Human papillomavirus-DNA loads in actinic keratoses exceed those in non-melanoma skin cancers. J Invest Dermatol 2005; 125:93-97.

[49] Yutsudo M, Hakura A. Human papillomavirus type 17 transcripts expressed in skin carcinoma tissue of a patient with epidermodysplasia verruciformis. Int J Cancer 1987; 39: 586-589.

[50] Haller K, Stubenrauch F, Pfister H. Differentiation-dependent transcription of the epidermodysplasia verruciformis-associated human papillomavirus type 5 in benign lesions. Virology 1995; 214 245-255.

[51] Purdie KJ, Surentheran T, Sterling JC, Bell L, McGregor JM, Proby CM, Harwood CA, Breuer J. Human papillomavirus gene expression in cutaneous squamous cell carcinomas from immunosuppressed and immunocompetent individuals. J Invest Dermatol 2005; 125 98-107.

[52] Dang C, Koehler A, Forschner T, Sehr P, Michael K, Pawlita M, Stockfleth E, Nindl I. E6/E7 expression of human papillomavirus types in cutaneous squamous cell dysplasia and carcinoma in immunosuppressed organ transplant recipients. Br J Dermatol 2006; 155 129-136.

[53] Cockayne EA. Inherited abnormalities of the skin and its appendages. London: Oxford University Press; 1933. p156.

[54] Rajagopalan K, Bahru J, Loo DS, Tay CH, Chin KN, Tan KK. Familial epidermodysplasia verruciformis of Lewandowsky and Lutz. Arch Dermatol 1972; 105 73-78.

[55] Sehgal VN, Luthra A, Bajaj P. Epidermodysplasia verruciformis: 14 members of a pedigree with an intriguing squamous cell carcinoma transformation. Int J Dermatol 2002; 41:500–503.

[56] Androphy EJ, Dvoretzky I, Lowy DR. X-linked inheritance of epidermodysplasia verruciformis: Genetic and virologic studies of a kindred. Arch Dermatol 1985; 121 864-868.

[57] Orth G. Genetics of epidermodysplasia verruciformis: insights into host defense against papillomaviruses. Semin Immunol 2006; 18 362-374.

[58] Ramoz N, Rueda LA, Bouadjar B, Favre M, Orth G. A susceptibility locus for epidermodysplasia verruciformis, an abnormal predisposition to infection with the oncogenic human papillomavirus type 5, maps to chromosome 17qter in a region containing a psoriasis locus. J Invest Dermatol 1999; 112 259-263.

[59] Aochi S, Nakanishi G, Suzuki N, Setsu N, Suzuki D, Aya K, Iwatsuki K. A novel homozygous mutation of the EVER1/TMC6 gene in a Japanese patient with epidermodysplasia verruciformis. Br J Dermatol 2007; 157 1265-1266.

[60] Gober MD, Rady PL, He Q, Tucker SB, Tyring SK, Gaspari AA. Novel homozygous frameshift mutation of EVER1 gene in an epidermodysplasia verruciformis patient. J Invest Dermatol 2007; 127 817-820.

[61] Rady PL, De Oliveira WR, He Q, Festa C, Rivitti EA, Tucker SB, Tyring SK. Novel homozygous nonsense TMC8 mutation detected in patients with epidermodysplasia verruciformis from a Brazilian family. Br J Dermatol 2007; 157 831-833.

[62] Sun XK, Chen JF, Xu AE. A homozygous nonsense mutation in the EVER2 gene leads to epidermodysplasia verruciformis. Clin Exp Dermatol 2005; 30 573-574.

[63] Tate G, Suzuki T, Kishimoto K, Mitsuya T. Novel mutations of EVER1/TMC6 gene in a Japanese patient with epidermodysplasia verruciformis. J Hum Genet 2004; 49(4) 223-225.

[64] Zuo YG, Ma D, Zhang Y, Qiao J, Wang B. Identification of a novel mutation and a genetic polymorphism of EVER1 gene in two families with epidermodysplasia verruciformis. J Dermatol Sci 2006 44(3) 153-159.

[65] Arnold AW, Burger B, Kump E, Rufle A, Tyring SK, Kempf W, Häusermann P, Itin PH. Homozygosity for the c.917A→T (p.N306I) polymorphism in the EVER2/TMC8 gene of two sisters with epidermodysplasia verruciformis Lewandowsky-Lutz originally described by Wilhelm Lutz. Dermatology 2011; 222(1) 81-86.

[66] Patel AS, Karagas MR, Pawlita M, Waterboer T, Nelson HH. Cutaneous human papillomavirus infection, the EVER2 gene and incidence of squamous cell carcinoma: a case-control study. Int J Cancer 2008; 122(10) 2377-2379.

[67] Berthelot C, Dickerson MC, Rady P, He Q, Niroomand F, Tyring SK, Pandya AG. Treatment of a patient with epidermodysplasia verruciformis carrying a novel EVER2 mutation with imiquimod. J Am Acad Dermatol 2007; 56(5) 882-886.

[68] Landini MM, Zavattaro E, Borgogna C, Azzimonti B, De Andrea M, Colombo E, Marenco F, Amantea A, Landolfo S, Gariglio M. Lack of EVER2 protein in two epidermodysplasia verruciformis patients with skin cancer presenting previously unreported homozygous genetic deletions in the EVER2 gene. J Invest Dermatol 2012; 132(4) 1305-1308.

[69] Akgül B, Köse O, Safali M, Purdie K, Cerio R, Proby C, Storey A. A distinct variant of Epidermodysplasia verruciformis in a Turkish family lacking EVER1 and EVER2 mutations. J Dermatol Sci 2007; 46(3) 214-216.

[70] Zavattaro E, Azzimonti B, Mondini M, De Andrea M, Borgogna C, Dell'Oste V, Ferretti M, Nicola S, Cappellano G, Carando A, Leigheb G, Landolfo S, Dianzani U, Gariglio M. Identification of defective Fas function and variation of the perforin gene in an epidermodysplasia verruciformis patient lacking EVER1 and EVER2 mutations. J Invest Dermatol 2008; 128(3) 732-735.

[71] McDermott DF, Gammon B, Snijders PJ, Mbata I, Phifer B, Howland Hartley A, Lee CC, Murphy PM, Hwang ST. Autosomal dominant epidermodysplasia verruciformis lacking a known EVER1 or EVER2 mutation. Pediatr Dermatol 2009; 26(3) 306-310.

[72] Lazarczyk M, Favre M. Role of Zn2+ ions in host-virus interactions. J Virol 2008; 82(23) 11486-11494.

[73] Lazarczyk M, Pons C, Mendoza JA, Cassonnet P, Jacob Y, Favre M. Regulation of cellular zinc balance as a potential mechanism of EVER-mediated protection against pathogenesis by cutaneous oncogenic human papillomaviruses. J Exp Med 2008; 205(1) 35-42.

Chapter 11

Maffucci Syndrome

Miki Tanioka

Additional information is available at the end of the chapter

http://dx.doi.org/10.5772/54570

1. Introduction

Maffucci syndrome is characterized by the presence of multiple enchondromas associated with multiple hemangiomas (figure 1). Enchondromas are common benign cartilage tumors of bone. They can occur as solitary lesions or as multiple lesions in enchondromatosis (Schwartz 1987, Kaplan 1993). When hemangiomata are associated, the condition is known as Maffucci syndrome (figure 2). The patients are normal at birth and the syndrome manifests during childhood and puberty. The enchondromas affect the extremities and their distribution is asymmetrical. The most common sites of enchondromas are the metacarpal bones and phalanges of the hands. The feet are less commonly afflicted. Clinical problems caused by enchondromas include skeletal deformity and the potential for malignant change to osteosarcoma (figure 3). The risk for sarcomatous degeneration of enchondromas, hemangiomas, or lymphangiomas is 15-30%. Maffucci syndrome is also associated with a higher risk of CNS, pancreatic, and ovarian malignancies (Ono 2012) (figure 4).

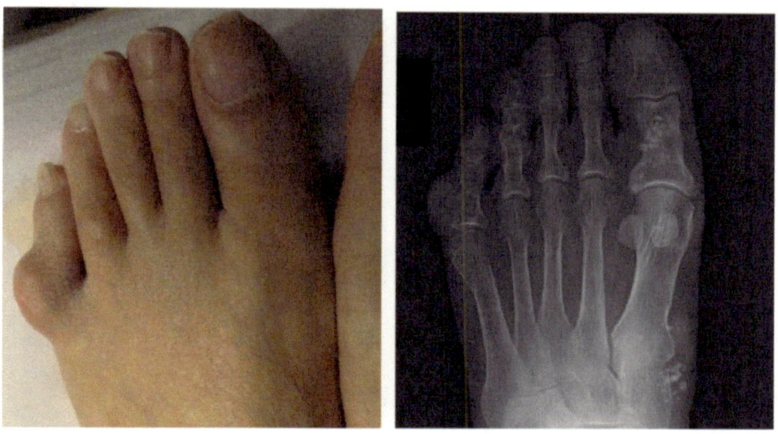

Figure 1. Multiple enchondromas

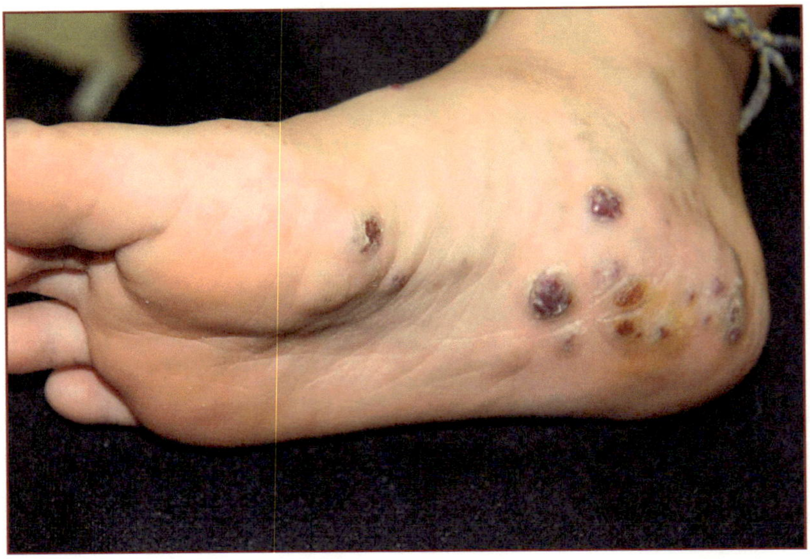

Figure 2. Multiple hemangioma on the sole

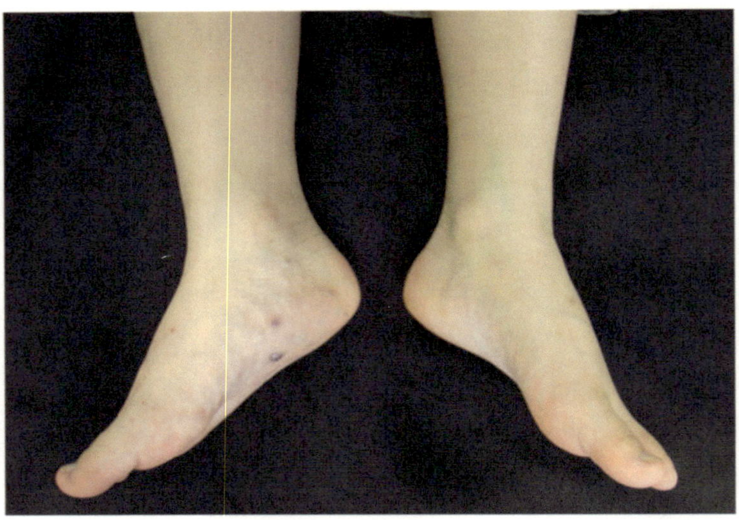

Figure 3. The differences of length and size of the legs are noted.

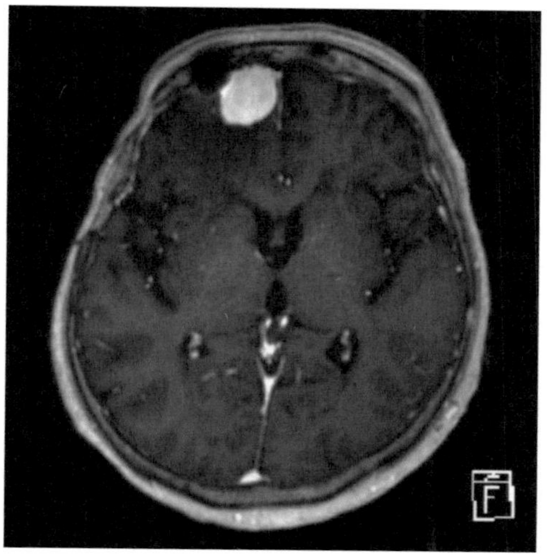

Figure 4. Brain tumor in a patient with Maffucci syndrome

2. Inheritance

Most cases of Maffucci syndrome have been sporadic and no specific hereditary form has been proven (Hakak and Azouz 1991).

It occurs in all races, and occurs in both sexes equally.

3. Cutaneous presentation of Maffucci syndrome

Multiple hemangiomas are presented as multiple nodules on the skin of the extremities, which looks like grapes (figure 2). However, the sites of hamangiomas are reported to be the colon and brain (Lee 1999). Multiple enchondromas present as a subcutaneous nodules fix to the underlining bones. Bleeding from the hemangiomas is clinically important and difficult to manage. Complete resection is usually impossible. Compression therapy is recommended.

4. Melecular genetics of Maffucci syndrome

The responsible genes for Maffucci syndrome have not been found. However, some studies were reported for multiple enchondromatosis.

In enchondromas and chondrosarcomas, mutations of the *PTHR1* gene was reported to be a candidate gene, however, subsequent studies could not confirm it (Hopyan 2002, Rozeman 2004).

Somatic heterozygous mutations in *IDH1* or *IDH2* were reported in enchondromas and spindle cell hemangiomas (Pansuriya 2011). Ten cases of 13 (77%) with Maffucci syndrome carried *IDH1* or *IDH2* mutations in their tumors. *IDH1* mutations in cartilage tumors were associated with hypermethylation and downregulated expression of several genes (Amary

2011). Mutations were absent in DNA isolated from the blood, muscle, or saliva of the subjects. Therefore, these mutations are believed to be somatic.

5. Management of Maffucci syndrome

Management entails careful examination and monitoring for malignant degenerations. Surgical interventions can correct or minimize deformities.

Compression therapy may be useful to control hemangiomas.

Author details

Miki Tanioka
Department of Dermatology, Graduate School of Medicine, Kyoto University, Shogoin-Kawara-cho, Sakyo-ku, Kyoto, Japan

6. References

Schwartz, H. S., Zimmerman, N. B., Simon, M. A., Wroble, R. R., Millar, E. A., Bonfiglio, M. The malignant potential of enchondromatosis. J. Bone Joint Surg. Am. 69: 269-274, 1987.

Kaplan, R. P., Wang, J. T., Amron, D. M., Kaplan, L. Maffucci's syndrome: two case reports with a literature review. J. Am. Acad. Derm. 29: 894-899, 1993.

Ono S, Tanizaki H, Fujisawa A, Tanioka M, Miyachi Y.Maffucci syndrome complicated with meningioma and pituitary adenoma.*Eur J Dermatol* 22(1):130-1, 2012.

Halal, F., Azouz, E. M. Generalized enchondromatosis in a boy with only platyspondyly in the father. Am. J. Med. Genet. 38: 588-592, 1991.

Lee, N. H., Choi, E. H., Choi, W. K., Lee, S. H., Ahn, S. K. Maffucci's syndrome with oral and intestinal haemangioma. (Letter) Brit. J. Derm. 140: 968-969, 1999.

Hopyan, S., Gokgoz, N., Poon, R., Gensure, R. C., Yu, C., Cole, W. G., Bell, R. S., Juppner, H., Andrulis, I. L., Wunder, J. S., Alman, B. A. A mutant PTH/PTHrP type I receptor in enchondromatosis. Nature Genet. 30: 306-310, 2002.

Rozeman, L. B., Sangiorgi, L., Briaire-de Bruijn, I. H., Mainil-Varlet, P., Bertoni, F., Cleton-Jansen, A. M., Hogendoorn, P. C. W., Bovee, J. V. M. G. Enchondromatosis (Ollier disease, Maffucci syndrome) is not caused by the PTHR1 mutation p.R150C. Hum. Mutat. 24: 466-473, 2004

Pansuriya, T. C., van Eijk, R., d'Adamo, P., van Ruler, M. A. J. H., Kuijjer, M. L., Oosting, J., Cleton-Jansen, A.-M., van Oosterwijk, J. G., Verbeke, S. L. J., Meijer, D., van Wezel, T., Nord, K. H., and 15 others. Somatic mosaic IDH1 and IDH2 mutations are associated with enchondroma and spindle cell hemangioma in Ollier disease and Maffucci syndrome. Nature Genet. 43: 1256-1261, 2011.

Amary, M. F., Damato, S., Halai, D., Eskandarpour, M., Berisha, F., Bonar, F., McCarthy, S., Fantin, V. R., Straley, K. S., Lobo, S., Aston, W., Green, C. L., Gale, R. E., Tirabosco, R., Futreal, A., Campbell, P., Presneau, N., Flanagan, A. M. Ollier disease and Maffucci syndrome are caused by somatic mosaic mutations of IDH1 and IDH2. Nature Genet. 43: 1262-1265, 2011.

Chapter 12

Nevoid Basal Cell Carcinoma Syndrome (NBCCS)

Miki Tanioka

Additional information is available at the end of the chapter

http://dx.doi.org/10.5772/54571

1. Introduction

Nevoid basal cell carcinoma syndrome (NBCCS) is characterized by the presence of multiple basal cell carcinomas associated with palmoplantar pits (Gorlin 1960). The patients are normal at birth and the syndrome manifests as palmoplantar pits in their early childhood. In their teens, odontogenic keratocysts (jaw cysts) develops and they are the first complain to visit hospitals (Evans 1993). Basal cell carcinomas (BCCs) present in their 40's, which is much earlier than sporadic BCCs. The other characteristic signs are bifid rib, calcification of the falx (Kimonis 1997).

NBCCS is associated with a higher risk of medulloblastoma, and ovarian malignancies (figures 1, 2, 3).

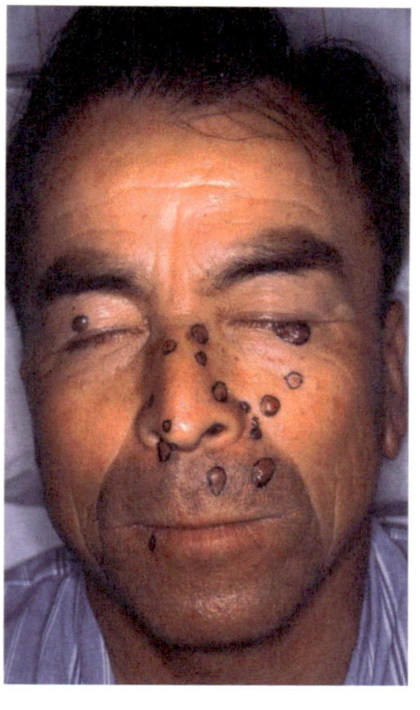

Figure 1. Multile BCCs on the face.

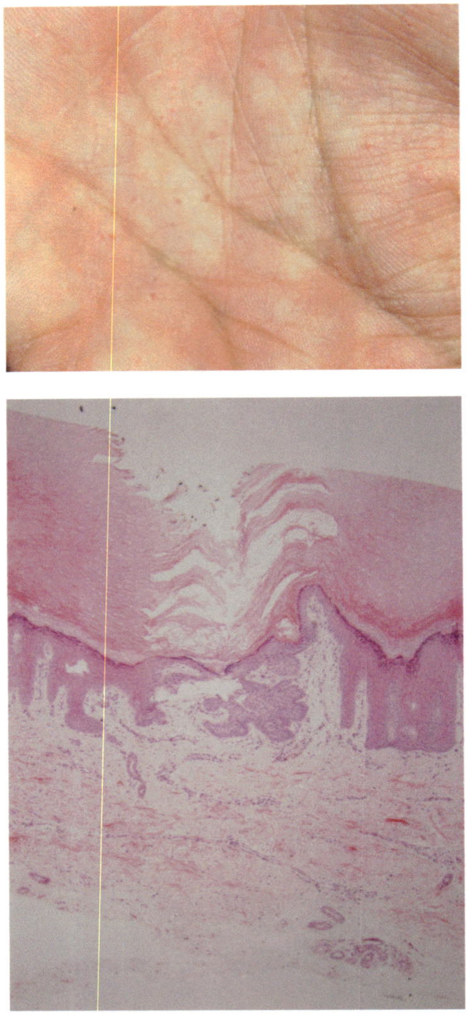

Figure 2. Palmar pits and its pathology.

2. Inheritance

Inheritance was autosomal dominant (Gorlin 1993). About 40% of cases represent a de novo mutation. It occurs in all races, and occurs in both sexes equally. The prevalence is reported to be 1 case per 56,000-164,000 population.

No genotype/phenotype relations have been reported.

3. Cutaneous presentation of NBCCS

Palmoplantar pits are the earliest clinical signs in their childhood. The keratinocytes under the pits are BCC-like, and its keratinization is abnormal, therefore the reduced stratified corneum looks like a pit.

Multiple basal cell carcinomas usually develops over their 40's. Usually sporadic BCC develops on the sun-exposed area in elderly people, especially on the face.

However, in NBCCS, BCC can develop on any areas of the body, which are not generally exposed to sunlight, such as the palms and soles of the feet and in younger people.

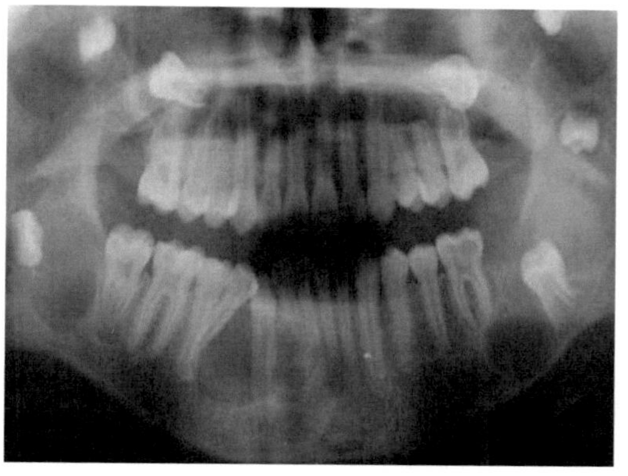

Figure 3. Multiple odontogenic keratocysts (jaw cysts) in the jaw.

4. Molecular genetics of NBCCS and its molecular mechanism

The responsible genes for NBCCS are the *PTCH1* gene on chromosome 9q22, the *PTCH2* gene on 1q32 and the *SUFU* gene on 10q24-q25 (Johnson 1996, Hahn 1996, Smyth 1999, Pastorino 2009). These genes mutations result in abnormalities in sonic hedgehog (SHH) signaling pathway components, which lead to the development of basal cell carcinomas. The sequence of *PTCH2* identities with 54 % of that of *PTCH1*. All three mammalian hedgehogs bind both receptors with similar affinity, so PTCH1 and PTCH2 cannot discriminate between the ligands.

No founder effects have been reported and almost all mutations are speculated to be *de novo*. No genotype/phenotype relations have been reported. Each person who has this syndrome is affected to a different degree, some having many more characteristics of the condition than others (Tanioka 2005).

Both PTCH1 and PTCH2 are coding a twelve transmembrane receptor whose lignad is sonic hedgehog (SHH)(Ingham 2011). SHH is a ~45kDa precursor and undergoes autocatalytic processing to produce an ~20kDa N-terminal signaling domain and a ~25kDa C-terminal domain with no known signaling role. SHH can signal in an autocrine fashion, affecting the cells in which it is produced.

In the absence of SHH, PTCH1 inhibits Smoothened (SMO), which is a downstream membrane protein in the SHH pathway (Taipale 2002). SMO is regulated by a small molecule, the cellular localization of which is controlled by PTCH (Strutt 2001).

The molecular mechanism is not fully understood, however, it should be associated with choresterol (Davies 2000). PTCH1 has a sterol sensing domain (SSD), which has been shown to be essential for suppression of Smo activity. In addition, PTCH1 has homology to Niemann-Pick disease, type C1 (NPC1) that is known to transport lipophilic molecules across a membrane. It is believed that PTCH regulates SMO by removing oxysterols from SMO. PTCH acts like a sterol pump and removes oxysterols that have been created by 7-dehydrocholesterol reductase. Upon binding of a SHH protein or a mutation in the SSD of PTCH the pump is turned off allowing oxysterols to accumulate around SMO.

The binding of SHH relieves SMO inhibition, leading to activation of the GLI transcription factors: the activators Gli1 and Gli2 and the repressor Gli3 (Shimokawa 2006). The sequence of molecular events that connect SMO to GLIs is poorly understood. However, in NBSSC, it is believed that activated Gli leads to the upregulated cell cycle of BCC cells (Epstein 1998). Recently, some drugs that blocks the SHH pathways have been developed and many clinical trials are undergoing.

5. Management of NBCCS

Management is careful examination and monitoring for malignant degenerations. Surgical interventions of jaw cysts can correct or minimize deformities. Surgical removal of basal cell carcinomas and medulloblastomas are recommended. Recently, a drug, vismodegib, which target the SMO are proved to be effective to control unresectable BCC and newly development of BCCs in NBCCS patients (Sekulic 2012, Tang 2012). Vismodegib is a new orally administered hedgehog-pathway inhibitor that produces objective responses in locally advanced and metastatic basal cellcarcinomas. Vismodegib reduces the basal-cell carcinoma tumor burden and blocks growth of new basal-cell carcinomas in patients with the basal-cell nevus syndrome. The adverse events associated with treatment led to discontinuation in over half of treated patients. Those included loss of taste, muscle cramps, hair loss, and weight loss.

Author details

Miki Tanioka
Department of Dermatology, Graduate School of Medicine, Kyoto University, Kyoto, Japan

6. References

Aleksandar Sekulic, M.D., Ph.D., Michael R. Migden, M.D., Anthony E. Oro, M.D., Ph.D., Luc Dirix, M.D., Ph.D., Karl D. Lewis, M.D., John D. Hainsworth, M.D., James A. Solomon, M.D., Ph.D., Simon Yoo, M.D., Sarah T. Arron, M.D., Ph.D., Philip A. Friedlander, M.D., Ph.D., Ellen Marmur, M.D., Charles M. Rudin, M.D., Ph.D., Anne Lynn S. Chang, M.D., Jennifer A. Low, M.D., Ph.D., Howard M. Mackey, Ph.D., Robert L. Yauch, Ph.D., Richard A. Graham, Ph.D., Josina C. Reddy, M.D., Ph.D., and Axel Hauschild, M.D. Efficacy and Safety of Vismodegib in Advanced Basal-Cell Carcinoma N Engl J Med 2012;366:2171-9.

Davies, J. P.; Chen, FW; Ioannou, YA (2000). "Transmembrane Molecular Pump Activity of Niemann-Pick C1 Protein". *Science* 290 (5500): 2295–8.

Epstein, Ervin H.; De Sauvage, Frederic J.; Xie, Jingwu; Murone, Maximilien; Luoh, Shiuh-Ming; Ryan, Anne; Gu, Qimin; Zhang, Chaohui et al. (1998). "Activating Smoothened mutations in sporadic basal-cell carcinoma". *Nature* 391 (6662): 90–2.

Evans, D. G. R., Ladusans, E. J., Rimmer, S., Burnell, L. D., Thakker, N., Farndon, P. A. Complications of the naevoid basal cell carcinoma syndrome: results of a population based study. J. Med. Genet. 30: 460-464, 1993.

Gorlin, R. J. From oral pathology to craniofacial genetics. Am. J. Med. Genet. 46: 317-334, 1993.

Gorlin, R. J., Goltz, R. W. Multiple nevoid basal-cell epithelioma, jaw cysts and bifid rib: a syndrome. New Eng. J. Med. 262: 908-912, 1960.

Hahn, H., Wicking, C., Zaphiropoulos, P. G., Gailani, M. R., Shanley, S., Chidambaram, A., Vorechovsky, I., Holmberg, E., Unden, A. B., Gillies, S., Negus, K., Smyth, I., Pressman, C., Leffell, D. J., Gerrard, B., Goldstein, A. M., Dean, M., Toftgard, R., Chenevix-Trench, G., Wainwright, B., Bale, A. E. Mutations of the human homolog of Drosophila patched in the nevoid basal cell carcinoma syndrome. Cell 85: 841-851, 1996.

Ingham, Philip W.; Nakano, Yoshiro; Seger, Claudia (2011). "Mechanisms and functions of Hedgehog signalling across the metazoa". *Nature Reviews Genetics* 12 (6): 393–406.

Jean Y. Tang, M.D., Ph.D., Julian M. Mackay-Wiggan, M.D., Michelle Aszterbaum, M.D., Robert L. Yauch, Ph.D., Joselyn Lindgren, M.S., Kris Chang, B.A., Carol Coppola, R.N., Anita M. Chanana, B.A., Jackleen Marji, M.D., Ph.D., David R. Bickers, M.D., and Ervin H. Epstein, Jr., M.D. Inhibiting the Hedgehog Pathway in Patients with the Basal-Cell Nevus Syndrome N Engl J Med 2012;366:2180-8.

Johnson, R. L., Rothman, A. L., Xie, J., Goodrich, L. V., Bare, J. W., Bonifas, J. M., Quinn, E. H., Myers, R. M., Cox, D. R., Epstein, E. H., Jr., Scott, M. P. Human homolog of patched, a candidate gene for the basal cell nevus syndrome. Science 272: 1668-1671, 1996.

Kimonis, V. E., Goldstein, A. M., Pastakia, B., Yang, M. L., Kase, R., DiGiovanna, J. J., Bale, A. E., Bale, S. J. Clinical manifestations in 105 persons with nevoid basal cell carcinoma syndrome. Am. J. Med. Genet. 69: 299-308, 1997.

Pastorino, L., Ghiorzo, P., Nasti, S., Battistuzzi, L., Cusano, R., Marzocchi, C., Garre, M. L., Clementi, M., Bianchi Scarra, G. Identification of a SUFU germline mutation in a family with Gorlin syndrome. Am. J. Med. Genet. 149A: 1539-1543, 2009.

Shimokawa, Takashi; Rahnama, Fahimeh; Lauth, Matthias; Finta, Csaba; Kogerman, Priit; Teglund, Stephan; Toftgård, Rune; Zaphiropoulos, Peter G. (2006). "Inhibition of GLI1 gene activation by Patched1" (//www.ncbi.nlm.nih.gov/pmc/articles/PMC1385998/) . *Biochemical Journal* 394 (Pt 1): 19–26.

Smyth, I., Narang, M. A., Evans, T., Heimann, C., Nakamura, Y., Chenevix-Trench, G., Pietsch, T., Wicking, C., Wainwright, B. J. Isolation and characterization of human Patched 2 (PTCH2), a putative tumour suppressor gene in basal cell carcinoma and medulloblastoma on chromosome 1p32. Hum. Molec. Genet. 8: 291-297, 1999.

Strutt, H.; Thomas, C.; Nakano, Y.; Stark, D.; Neave, B.; Taylor, A.M.; Ingham, P.W. (2001). "Mutations in the sterol-sensing domain of Patched suggest a role for vesicular trafficking in Smoothened regulation". *Current Biology* 11 (8): 608–13.

Taipale, J.; Cooper, M. K.; Maiti, T.; Beachy, P. A. (2002). "Patched acts catalytically to suppress the activity of Smoothened". *Nature* 418 (6900): 892–7.

Tanioka M, Takahashi K, Kawabata T, Kosugi S, Murakami KI, Miyachi Y, Nishigori C and Iizuka T Germline mutations of the *PTCH* gene in Japanese patients with nevoid basal cell carcinoma syndrome. *Arch Dermatol Res* 296(7): 303-308, 2005.

Chapter 13

Multiple Cutaneous and Uterine Leiomyomatosis

Teruhiko Makino

Additional information is available at the end of the chapter

http://dx.doi.org/10.5772/53601

1. Introduction

Multiple cutaneous and uterine leiomyomatosis (MCUL: OMIM 150800), which is also known as Reed syndrome, is an autosomal dominant disorder in which benign skin tumors arising from the arrector pili muscle and uterine fibroids typically develop in the third and fourth decades [1, 2]. Reed *et al* first reported on two families in which members of successive generations demonstrated cutaneous leiomyomas, uterine leiomyomas, and/or leiomyosarcomas in 1973 [3]. A small population of families with MCUL has also been reported to demonstrate clusters of renal cancer, either manifesting as type 2 papillary renal cell carcinoma or renal collecting duct cancer. This latter disease variant is referred to as hereditary leiomyomatosis and renal cell cancer (HLRCC: OMIM 605839) [4, 5]. Heterozygous germline mutations in the *fumarate hydratase (FH, fumarase)* gene (MIM 136850) mapped on chromosome 1q42.3-q43 are detected in both MCUL and HLRCC and many different mutations have been reported in the *FH* gene [6, 7]. The *FH* gene encodes the fumarate hydratase (FH) enzyme, that catalyzes the conversion of fumarate to malate as part of the TCA cycle in the mitochondrial matrix. This chapter will initially explain the clinical manifestations and etiology of MCUL/HLRCC based on the data from previous reports. The structure and fundamental function of the FH protein, *FH* gene mutation and the relation between alteration of FH protein and tumorigenesis in MCUL/HLRCC will be addressed. Finally, the diagnosis and treatments of MCUL/HLRCC is also explained.

2. Clinical manifestations

2.1. Cutaneous leiomyomas

The most prominent feature of MCUL/HLRCC is the occurrence of solitary or multiple cutaneous leiomyomas, which appear as firm skin-colored or pink-brown papules or nodules up to 2cm in diameter and are often associated with pain (Figure 1) [1]. The distribution of skin lesions shows approximately equal numbers of patients with clustered leiomyomas only, scattered leiomyomas only, and a combination of clustered and scattered lesions. Clustered lesions are most common on the trunk, followed by the lower limb(s), upper limb(s), and head and neck. Scattered lesions are most often found on the the upper limb(s), followed by the trunk, lower limb(s), and head and neck. A small proportion of patients have symmetrically distributed or unilaterally distributed lesions. In addition, band-like or type 2 segmental manifestations have also been reported [8]. Skin leiomyomas are reported to develop at a mean age of 24.1 years (median, 25 years; range, 9-45 years), although the mean ages of symptom onset and diagnosis are 31.4 and 36.6 years, respectively. These tumors seem to remain benign. Only two cases of skin leiomyosarcoma in association with an *FH* germline mutation have been reported [9, 10]. A histological examination shows that all cutaneous leiomyomas are pilar lesions occurring superficially in the dermis (Figure 2). They were thought to originate from the pili arrector muscles of the hair follicle. Smooth muscle fiber bundles composed of eosinophilic cytoplasm with elongated blunt-ended nuclei with little or no waviness are interspersed with collagen within the dermis [11]. An immunohistochemical study revealed the presence of markers of smooth muscle differentiation, such as desmin and actin (Figure 3). Estrogen and progesterone receptors are negative in cutaneous leiomyomas, although these are positive in uterine leiomyomas [12].

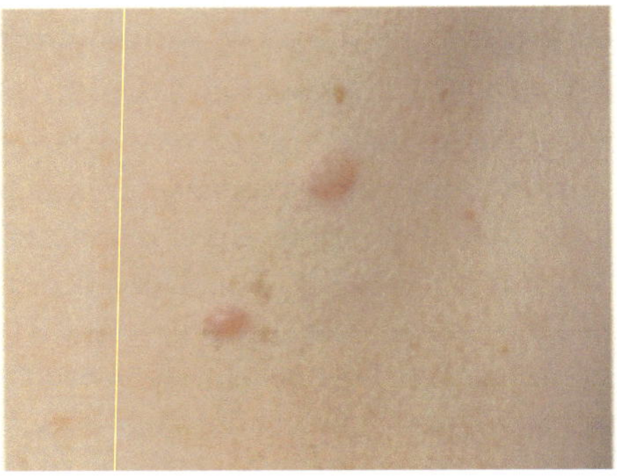

Figure 1. Clinical presentation of cutaneous leiomyoma. Redish nodules up to 2cm in diametar.

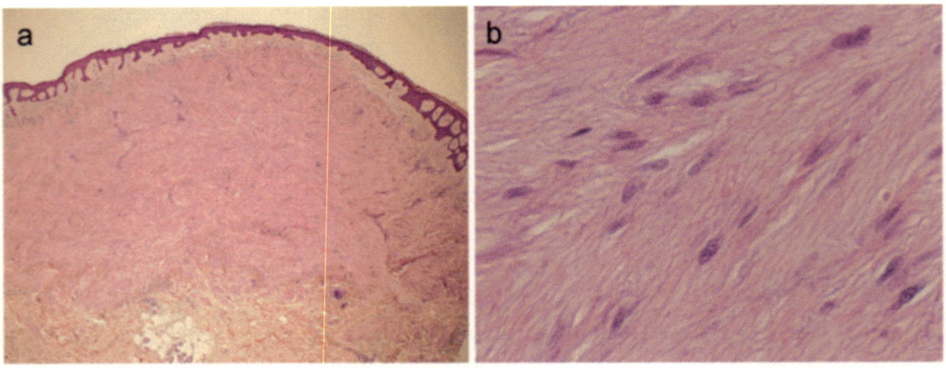

Figure 2. a. Histological examination of cutaneous leiomyoma shows interlacing fasicles of the smooth muscle cells within the dermis (hamtoxylin and eosin staining, original modification x40). b. Tumor cells are composed of eosinophilic cytoplasm with wlogated blunt-ended nuclei. There were no atypia or mitosis present (hematoxylin and eosin staining, original modification x400)

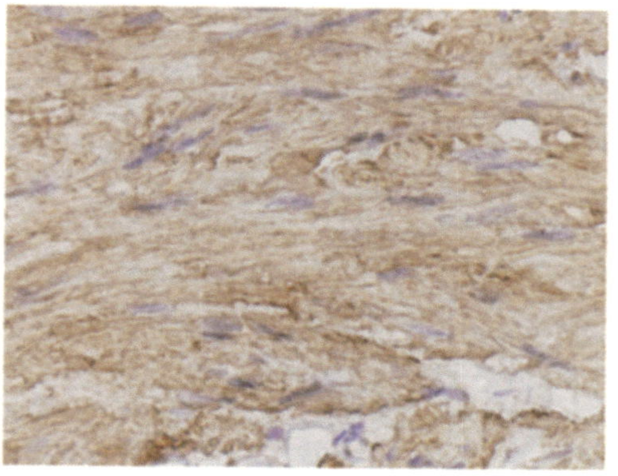

Figure 3. Immunohistological findings of cutaneous leiomyioma. Tumor cells were positive for smooth muscle actin immunostaining (original magnification x400)

2.2. Uterine fibroids

Uterine fibroids (leiomyomas) are benign tumors that develop from the smooth muscle cells of the uterus. The common symptoms including irregular menses, menorrhagia, pain and defects in the reproductive functions, show no difference between uterine fibroids in MCUL/HLRCC and those of sporadic cases; however, the clinical features in MCUL/HLRCC are different from those in sporadic cases. Many uterine fibroids are observed in MCUL/HLRCC and the size of tumors in MCUL/HLRCC is larger than that of sporadic cases [9, 10]. The mean age at the time of diagnosis of uterine fibroids with MCUL/HLRCC is around 30 years (range 18-53) and it is approximately 10 years before the diagnosis in sporadic cases. Most female patients (79-100%) with an *FH* gene mutation are affected with uterine fibroids [10,13]. The association of the generally rare uterine leiomyosarcoma with the syndrome has also been suggested; however, the biological behavior of the uterine tumors in HLRCC has remained unclear [14].

2.3. Renal cell carcinoma

Renal cell carcinoma (RCC) is a tumor arising from the epithelium of the renal tubules. RCC can be classified into morphological subtypes including clear cell, papillary, chromophobe and collecting duct carcinoma [15, 16]. The most frequent type of RCC in HLRCC is a type 2 papillary RCC [17]. The tumor histologically shows a papillary growth pattern. The tumor cells show a large nucleus with a prominent eosinophilic nucleus surrounded by a clear halo. Cystic components also seem to be typical findings [18, 19]. These features are suggested to be characteristic of a RCC in HLRCC. In addition, collecting duct tumors, oncocytic tumors and clear cell tumors have also been reported [9, 10, 18, 20]. An immunohistochemical study of RCC in HLRCC showed the absence of the cytokeratin (CK) 7 and the expression of UEA-a protein. In addition, the absence of mucin, CK20 and CD10 is considered to be typical of the tumors [19, 21]. RCC in HLRCC is commonly solitary and unilateral. RCC is found in about 20-25% of the *FH* gene mutation positive families [22, 23].

Up to 32 and 50% of the North America and Finnish families, respectively, show the RCC phenotype [9, 10, 18] The mean age at the time of RCC diagnosis is 42 and 44 years in Finnish and North American HLRCC families, respectively. Approximately half cases of the RCC in HLRCC are detected in individuals younger than 40 years, many even less than 30 years [9, 20, 24]. The youngest of the RCC patients was 11 years old when diagnosed [24]. Importantly, HLRCC-associated renal cancers are very aggressive and can metastasize even though the primary tumor is small. Most reported patients die within 5 years after diagnosis creating a challenge for surveillance and treatment practices [9, 19, 25]. Therefore, annual pelvic/abdominal MRI starting from the age of 18 is considered to be effective practice, especially for individuals with a familial history of RCC. In addition, benign kidney cysts frequently develop in the carriers of *FH* gene mutation in comparison to individuals less than 40 years of age in the general population. Such cyst formation is suggested to result from an increased cell proliferation due to the activation of the hypoxia pathway and it has also been postulated to represent premalignant lesions [26, 27].

2.4. Fumarate hydratase

FH gene is located in the chromosomal region 1q42.1. It contains 10 exons and generates a transcript of 1.5 kb [28,29]. There is a mitochondria localization signal in the first exon. *FH* gene encodes two isoforms of the fumarate hydratase (FH) enzyme. The mitochondrial isoform of FH is one of the enzymes of the tricarboxylic acid cycle (TCA cycle, Kreb's cycle), which is a part of cellular respiration, the aerobic step of energy production (Figure 4). The active form of FH protein is a homotetramer with two substrate-binding sites [13] and it catalyzes the conversion of fumarate to malate in the mitochondrial matrix. In contrast, the function of the cytosolic FH isoform is thought to be involved in the fumarate and amino acid metabolism [30]. Previous studies suggest that some of the FH protein is translocated back to the cytosol from the mitochondria by removal of the mitochondrial localization signal [31].

Heterozygous germline mutations in *FH* gene were linked with both MCUL and HLRCC [6, 32]. Biallelic inactivation of FH is observed in associated tumors; therefore, FH is considered to be a tumor suppressor based on the Knudsen's two-hit hypothesis.

2.5. Mutations in *FH* gene

Approximately 100 different mutations have been reported in the *FH* gene according to the online *FH* variant database [22]. Missense, nonsense, frameshift, insertion, and splice-site mutations have been found in the *FH* gene. The majority (~58%) of these germline mutations are missense with the remaining being nonsense (~11%), and frameshift (~11%) mutations, located along the entire length of the *FH* gene coding region. Nonsense mutations result in the absence of FH or formation of a truncated FH protein product that is functionally inactive. Most of the heterozygous missense mutations are found in the looped regions of FH with important roles in forming the homotetramer according to the crystal structure of the *E.coli* fumarase C, which is useful in models for predicting the effect of missense

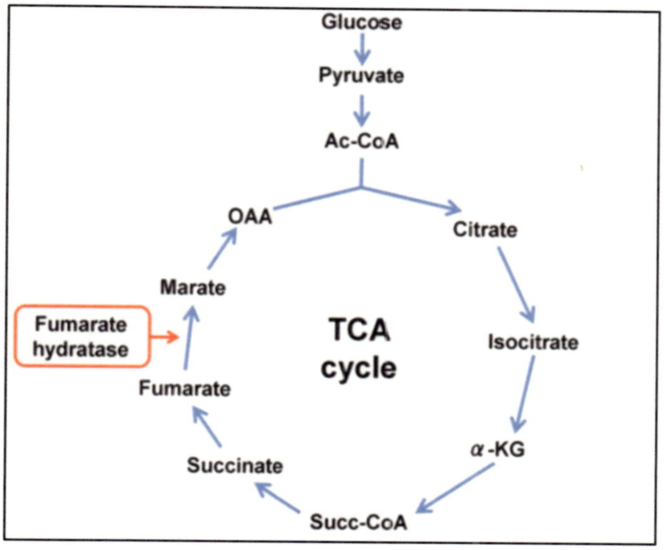

Figure 4. TCA cycle. Ac-CoA, acetyl coenzyme A; α-KG, α-ketoglurarase; Succ-CoA, succinyl coenzyme A; OOA, oxaloacetate.

mutations on human FH [33]. These missense mutations paradoxically cause marked reduction in the FH enzyme activity in comparison to truncated mutations [8, 13]. In addition, a hypothesis of the dominant negative effect of missense mutations has also been reported [34]. There appears to be no specific genotype-phenotype correlation with regard to which combination of these tumors develops in MCUL/HLRCC [32]. However, cases with RCC in HLRCC are mainly found in Finnish and North American families. This suggests that either environmental or additional genetic factors might be related to the induction of the malignant phenotype [2, 4-6, 10, 18]. Several other tumors have also been reported In the *FH* gene mutation carriers. However, biallelic inactivation of the *FH* gene was detected in only three cases of breast cancer, one case of bladder cancer, two cases of adult Leydig cell tumors and one case of adrenocortical hyperplastic lesion in Cushing syndrome [18, 35, 36]. The significance of *FH* gene mutation in the development of these tumors is still unclear although the *FH* gene defect might be involved in the tumorigenesis. In addition, biallelic *FH* germline mutations cause a rare recessive syndrome named FH deficiency (FHD or fumaric aciduria, MIM 606813), characterized by severe neurological symptoms such as psychomotor retardation, muscular hypotonia and microcephaly [37, 38].Dramatic reduction of the FH enzyme activity in a patient's tissues results in a metabolic crisis causing death commonly as an infant.

2.6. Molecular mechanism of MCUL/HLRCC tumorigenesis

Individuals with MCUL/HLRCC inherit one loss-of function allele and somatically lose the other allele in the tumor. The inherited *FH* gene mutations severely reduce enzyme activity, causing the tumors to accumulate high levels of fumarate [10]. Both loss of heterozygosity (LOH) and point mutations as second hits have been observed as this mechanism [5, 39].

Therefore, the *FH* gene is thought to act as a tumor suppressor gene [4]. However, the *FH* gene is not a typical tumor suppressor gene with a distinct anti-proliferative role, but rather its loss leads to more complex consequences. One of the broadly studied mechanisms is the so-called "pseudohypoxia" pathway referring to the induction of the hypoxia inducible factor 1 (HIF1) and its downstream targets under normoxic condition. HIF1 is a heterodimeric transcription factor formed by the HIF1α and HIF1β subunit. The proteosomal degradation of the HIF1α subunit is important for HIF1 regulation when molecular oxygen is available. HIF1 promotes adaptation of cells to non-physiological conditions when oxygen tension is low, by inducing anaerobic glycolysis as an alternative phosphorylation, and by inducing vascularization to facilitate the oxygen and nutrient supply into hypoxic tissues [40]. Fumarate, the substrate of FH, is shown to accumulate into the cytoplasm of cells and cause stabilization of HIF1 by inhibiting α-ketoglutarate (α-KG) dependent dioxygenase in MUCL/HLRCC tumors because of an FH defect [41-44]. The stabilized HIF1 plays a role as an activator in vascularization, glycolysis and glucose transport, which are significant pathways for promoting tumor growth [45]. Furthermore, FH deficiency precludes tumor cells from generating several of the TCA cycle intermediates, including malate, oxaloacetate and citrate, through conventional oxidative metabolism. [46, 47]. Human FH-deficient renal carcinoma cells redirect part of the TCA cycle, to compensate for this. This pathway appears to be a robust mechanism allowing cells to maintain growth during impaired oxidative metabolism, because it is also observed in human cancer cell lines with a mutation in the electron transport chain or in the Von Hippel-Lindau tumor suppressor, and in cells subjected to hypoxia, all of which negatively impact oxygen-dependent mitochondrial enzymes [48-51]. In addition, high levels of fumarate can induce aberrant patterns of gene expression. The electrophilic properties of fumarate allow it to modify cysteine residues on cellular proteins, producing an S-(2-succinyl)cysteine adduct in a Michael addition reaction termed succination [52]. Succination impairs protein function. Fumarate-mediated succination of Kelch-like ECH-associated protein 1 (Keap1) elicits an nuclear factor E2-related factor 2 (Nrf2) response In cells with FH deficiency, maintaining constitutively high expression of Nrf2 targets [53-55]. One of these targets is *HMOX1,* which encodes the enzyme required for heme degradation in FH-deficient cells, thus suggesting that fumarate-dependent suppression of Keap1 may promote cell survival, although the role the Keap1/Nrf2 system plays in tumorigenesis is unclear. Therefore, fumarate-mediated suppression of Keap1 may contribute to tumor development in the setting of FH deficiency.

2.7. Diagnosis

No diagnostic criteria for MUUL/HLRCC have been established; however, practical criteria for the clinical diagnosis of MUUL/HLRCC have been proposed [56]. Multiple cutaneous leiomyoma which is histologically confirmed is proposed as a major criterion. The minor criteria included uterine fibroids, papillary type 2 RCC or positive familial history. A molecular genetic analysis should be conducted to confirm the diagnosis when the clinical features are suggestive of MCUL/HLRCC. Direct sequencing of the *FH* gene cording region is commonly performed as a genetic analysis. This analysis detects underlying genetic alterations in about 90% of the suggestive MCUL/HLRCC cases [9, 10, 20, 57]. The possibility of exon or whole gene deletion is suspected If no mutation is detected in the *FH* gene, in spite of the fact that either patient's symptoms or familial history is strongly suggestive of UCML/HLRCC. The detection of possible copy-number changes in the *FH* gene might be useful in such case, by using additional methods such as multiplex ligation-dependent probe amplification [56, 58].

3. Treatment and management

3.1. Cutaneous leiomyomas and uterine fibroids

Cutaneous leiomyomas are commonly benign, and thus, the treatment for these tumors may be only improvement of cosmetic and pain related complications. Surgical excision is usually performed for the solitary tumors. The multiple painful lesions are generally treated with medications, such as nitoglycerol, calcium channel blockers, alpha-adrenoreceptor blockers, which have been reported to be occasionally successful to relieve pain [8]. Surgical approaches including hysterectomy are typically needed for uterine fibroids, based on the number and size of the tumors and the severity of the symptoms caused by the tumors [13, 57]. Furthermore, myomectomy, uterine artery embolization or pharmaceutical treatment with gonadotropin-releasing hormone agonist is also performed as an optional treatment for uterine fibroids.

3.2. Renal cell carcinoma

RCCs commonly acquires metastatic potential after exceeding the size of 3-7 cm [59]. Renal lesions can be observed until they reach the size of 3 cm, at which point they should be removed, and nephron sparing surgery usually appropriate [60]. However, RCC in HLRCC is thought to differ from sporadic RCCs because they are often metastatic at presentation even if the size of tumor is less than 1 cm. Therefore, tumors in HLRCC are recommended to be excised with radical surgery immediately [15, 59, 60]. Sorafenib and sunitinib, which are inhibitors of receptor tyrosine kinases activated by HIF1 targets such as VEGF, PDGF and TNF-α, have been used in the treatment of sporadic papillary RCC with varying success. These treatments are specific targeted pharmaceutical approaches. However, Information regarding the specific response of HLRCC associated tumors to these molecules is not available.

4. Conclusion

MCUL/HLRCC is a syndrome predisposing the *FH* gene mutation carriers mainly to benign tumors including cutaneous leiomyomas and uterine fibroids. Furthermore, renal cell carcinomas are also found in a subset of the HLRCC families and these are very aggressive in nature as small lesions. Therefore, appropriate surveillance with diagnostic examination for uterine and diseases is warranted in rare cases of multiple, biopsy-proven cutaneous lesions. Genetic analysis of the *FH* gene should be performed in all cases of suspected or confirmed disease. Genetic counseling is also recommended for other family members of the patient's family. Identification of the syndrome and its tumorigenic mechanisms has provided new insight in MCUL/HLRCC.

Author details

Teruhiko Makino
Department of Dermatology, Graduate School of Medicine and Pharmaceutical Sciences, University of Toyama, Toyama, Japan

5. References

[1] Garcia Muret MP, Pujol RM, Alomer A et al. Familial leiomyomatosis cutis et uteri (Reed's syndrome). Arch Dermatol Res 1988; 280: S29-32.

[2] Alam NA, Bevan S, Churchman M et al. Localization of a gene (MCUL1) for multiple cutaneous leiomyomata and uterine fibroids to chromosome 1q42.3-q43. Am J Hum Genet 2001; 68:1264–1269

[3] Reed WB, Walker R, Horowitz R. Cutaneous leiomyomata with uterine leiomyomata. Acta Derm Venereol 1973; 53:409–416

[4] Kiuru M, Launonen V, Hietala M et al. Familial cutaneous leiomyomatosis is a two-hit condition associated with renal cell cancer of characteristic histopathology. Am J Pathol 2001; 159: 825–829

[5] Launonen V, Vierimaa O, Kiuru M et al (2001) Inherited susceptibility to uterine leiomyomas and renal cell cancer. Proc Natl Acad Sci USA 98:3387–3392

[6] Tomlinson IP, Alam NA, Rowan AJ et al. Germline mutations in FH predispose to dominantly inherited uterine fibroids, skin leiomyomata and papillary renal cell cancer. Nat Genet 2002; 30: 406–410

[7] Badeloe S, van Geest AJ, van Marion AM et al. Absence of fumarate hydratase mutation in a family with cutaneous leiomyosarcoma and renal cancer. Int J Dermatol 2008; 47(Suppl 1): 18–20

[8] Ritzmann S, Hanneken S, Neumann NJ et al. Type 2 segmental manifestation of cutaneous leiomyomatosis in four unrelated women with additional uterine leiomyomas (Reed's syndrome). Dermatology 2006; 212: 84–87

[9] Toro JR, Nickerson ML, Wei MH et al. Mutations in the fumarate hydratase gene cause hereditary leiomyomatosis and renal cell cancer in families in North America. Am J Hum Genet 2003; 73:95–106

[10] Wei MH, Toure O, Glenn GM et al. Novel mutations in FH and expansion of the spectrum of phenotypes expressed in families with hereditary leiomyomatosis and renal cell cancer. J Med Genet 2006; 43: 18–27

[11] Kilpatrick SE, Mentzel T, Fletcher CD. Leiomyoma of deep soft tissue. Clinicopathologic analysis of a series. Am J Surg Pathol 1994; 18: 576–582.

[12] McGinley KM, Bryant S, Kattine AA, et al. Cutaneous leiomyomas lack estrogen and progesterone receptor immunoreactivity. J Cutan Pathol 1997; 24: 241–245.

[13] Alam NA, Barclay E, Rowan AJ et al. Clinical features of multiple cutaneous and uterine leiomyomatosis: an underdiagnosed tumor syndrome. Arch Dermatol 2005; 141: 199–206

[14] D'Angelo E, Prat J. Uterine sarcomas: a review. Gynecol Oncol 2010; 116: 131–139

[15] Cohen HT, McGovern FJ. Renal-cell carcinoma. N Engl J Med 2005; 353:2477–2490

[16] Eble JN, Sauter G, Epstein JI, Sesterhenn IA (ed.) World Health Organization classification of tumours: pathology & genetics of tumours of the urinary system and male genital organs. Lyon: IARC Press; 2004

[17] Delahunt B, Eble JN. Papillary renal cell carcinoma: a clinicopathologic and immunohistochemical study of 105 tumors. Mod Pathol 1997; 10: 537–544

[18] Lehtonen HJ. Molecular and clinical characteristics of tricarboxylic acid cycle-associated tumors. Dissertation: University of Helsinki; 2008

[19] Merino MJ, Torres-Cabala C, Pinto P et al. The morphologic spectrum of kidney tumors in hereditary leiomyomatosis and renal cell carcinoma (HLRCC) syndrome. Am J Surg Pathol 2007; 31: 1578–1585

[20] Alam NA, Rowan AJ, Wortham NC et al. Genetic and functional analyses of FH mutations in multiple cutaneous and uterine leiomyomatosis, hereditary leiomyomatosis and renal cancer, and fumarate hydratase deficiency. Hum Mol Genet 2003; 12: 1241–1252

[21] Lehtonen HJ, Kiuru M, Ylisaukko-Oja SK et al. Increased risk of cancer in patients with fumarate hydratase germline mutation. J Med Genet 2006; 43: 523–526

[22] Bayley JP, Launonen V, Tomlinson IP. The FH mutation database: an online database of fumarate hydratase mutations involved in the MCUL (HLRCC) tumor syndrome and congenital fumarase deficiency. BMC Med Genet 2008; 9: 20

[23] Koski TA. Molecular genetic background of tumours in hereditary leiomyomatosis and renal cell cancer syndrome. Dissertation: University of Helsinki; 2010

[24] Alrashdi I, Levine S, Paterson J et al. Hereditary leiomyomatosis and renal cell carcinoma: very early diagnosis of renal cancer in a paediatric patient. Fam Cancer 2010; 9: 239–243

[25] Grubb RL 3rd, Franks ME, Toro J et al. Hereditary leiomyomatosis and renal cell cancer: a syndrome associated with an aggressive form of inherited renal cancer. J Urol 2007; 177: 2074–2079

[26] Pollard PJ, Spencer-Dene B, Shukla D et al. Targeted inactivation of fh1 causes proliferative renal cyst development and activation of the hypoxia pathway. Cancer Cell 2007; 11: 311–319

[27] Mandriota SJ, Turner KJ, Davies DR et al. HIF activation identifies early lesions in VHL kidneys: evidence for site-specific tumor suppressor function in the nephron. Cancer Cell 2002; 1: 459–468

[28] Kinsella BT, Doonan S. Nucleotide sequence of a cDNA coding for mitochondrial fumarase from human liver. Biosci Rep 1986; 6: 921–929

[29] Tolley E, Craig I. Presence of two forms of fumarase (Fumarate Hydratase E.C. 4.2.1.2) in mammalian cells: immunological characterization and genetic analysis in somatic cell hybrids. Confirmation of the assignment of a gene necessary for the enzyme expression to human chromosome 1. Biochem Genet 1975; 13: 867–883

[30] Weaver TM, Levitt DG, Donnelly MI, et al. The multisubunit active site of fumarase C from Escherichia coli. Nat Struct Biol 1995; 2: 654-662.

[31] Sass E, Karniely S, Pines O. Folding of fumarase during mitochondrial import determines its dual targeting in yeast. J Biol Chem 2003; 278: 45109–45116

[32] Badeloe S, van Geel M, van Steensel MA et al. Diffuse and segmental variants of cutaneous leiomyomatosis: novel mutations in the fumarate hydratase gene and review of the literature. Exp Dermatol 2006; 15: 735–741

[33] Alam NA, Olpin S, Rowan A, et al: Missense mutation in Fumarate Hydratase in Multiple Cutaneous and Uterine Leiomyomatosis and Renal Cell Cancer. J Mol Diagn 2005; 7: 437-443.

[34] Lorenzato A, Olivero M, Perro M et al. A cancer-predisposing "hot spot" mutation of the fumarase gene creates a dominant negative protein. Int J Cancer 2008; 122: 947–951

[35] Matyakhina L, Freedman RJ, Bourdeau I et al. Hereditary leiomyomatosis associated with bilateral, massive, macronodular adrenocortical disease and atypical Cushing syndrome: a clinical and molecular genetic investigation. J Clin Endocrinol Metab 2005; 90: 3773–3779

[36] Carvajal-Carmona LG, Alam NA, Pollard PJ et al. Adult leydig cell tumors of the testis caused by germline fumarate hydratase mutations. J Clin Endocrinol Metab 2006; 91: 3071–3075

[37] Zinn AB, Kerr DS, Hoppel CL. Fumarase deficiency: a new cause of mitochondrial encephalomyopathy. N Engl J Med 1986; 315: 469–475

[38] Deschauer M, Gizatullina Z, Schulze A et al. Molecular and biochemical investigations in fumarase deficiency. Mol Genet Metab 2006; 88: 146–152

[39] Kiuru M, Lehtonen R, Arola J et al. Few FH mutations in sporadic counterparts of tumor types observed in hereditary leiomyomatosis and renal cell cancer families. Cancer Res 2002; 62: 4554–4557

[40] Semenza GL. Oxygen homeostasis. Wiley Interdiscip Rev Syst Biol Med 2010; 2: 336–361

[41] Pollard PJ, Briere JJ, Alam NA et al. Accumulation of Krebs cycle intermediates and over-expression of HIF1alpha in tumours which result from germline FH and SDH mutations. Hum Mol Genet 2005; 14: 2231–2239

[42] Isaacs JS, Jung YJ, Mole DR et al. HIF overexpression correlates with biallelic loss of fumarate hydratase in renal cancer: novel role of fumarate in regulation of HIF stability. Cancer Cell 2005; 8: 143–153

[43] MacKenzie ED, Selak MA, Tennant DA et al. Cell-permeating alpha-ketoglutarate derivatives alleviate pseudohypoxia in succinate dehydrogenase-deficient cells. Mol Cell Biol 2007; 27: 3282–3289

[44] Pan Y, Mansfield KD, Bertozzi CC et al. Multiple factors affecting cellular redox status and energy metabolism modulate hypoxia-inducible factor prolyl hydroxylase activity in vivo and in vitro. Mol Cell Biol 2007; 27: 912–925

[45] Ashrafian H, O'Flaherty L, Adam J et al. Expression profiling in progressive stages of fumarate-hydratase deficiency: the contribution of metabolic changes to tumorigenesis. Cancer Res 2010; 70: 9153–9165

[46] Shanware NP, Mullen AR, DeBerardinis RJ et al. Glutamine: pleiotropic roles in tumor growth and stress resistance. J Mol Med (Berl) 2011; 89: 229–236

[47] DeBerardinis RJ, Cheng T. Q's next: the diverse functions of glutamine in metabolism, cell biology and cancer. Oncogene 2010; 29: 313–324

[48] Wise DR, Ward PS, Shay JE et al. Hypoxia promotes isocitrate dehydrogenase-dependent carboxylation of alpha-ketoglutarate to citrate to support cell growth and viability. Proc. Natl. Acad. Sci. U.S.A. 2011; 108: 19611–19616

[49] Mullen AR, Wheaton WW, Jin ES et al. Reductive carboxylation supports growth in tumour cells with defective mitochondria. Nature 2012; 481: 385–388

[50] Metallo CM, Gameiro PA, Bell EL et al. Reductive glutamine metabolism by IDH1 mediates lipogenesis under hypoxia. Nature 2012; 481: 380–384

[51] Scott DA, Richardson AD, Filipp FV et al. Comparative metabolic flux profiling of melanoma cell lines: beyond the Warburg effect. J Biol Chem 2011; 286: 42626–42634

[52] Alderson NL, Wang Y, Blatnik M et al. S-(2-Succinyl) cysteine: a novel chemical modification of tissue proteins by a Krebs cycle intermediate. Arch Biochem Biophys 2006; 450: 1–8

[53] Ooi A, Wong JC, Petillo D et al. An antioxidant response phenotype shared between hereditary and sporadic type 2 papillary renal cell carcinoma. Cancer Cell 2011; 20: 511–523

[54] Adam J, Hatipoglu E, O'Flaherty L et al. Renal cyst formation in Fh1-deficient mice is independent of the Hif/Phd pathway: roles for fumarate in KEAP1 succination and Nrf2 signaling. Cancer Cell 2011; 20: 524–537

[55] Bardella C, El-Bahrawy M, Frizzell N et al. Aberrant succination of proteins in fumarate hydratase-deficient mice and HLRCC patients is a robust biomarker of mutation status. J Pathol 2011; 225: 4–11

[56] Smit DL, Mensenkamp AR, Badeloe S et al. Hereditary leiomyomatosis and renal cell cancer in families referred for fumarate hydratase germline mutation analysis. Clin Genet 2011; 79: 49-59

[57] Stewart L, Glenn GM, Stratton P et al. Association of germline mutations in the fumarate hydratase gene and uterine fibroids in women with hereditary leiomyomatosis and renal cell cancer. Arch Dermatol 2008; 144: 1584–1592

[58] Ahvenainen T, Lehtonen HJ, Lehtonen R et al. Mutation screening of fumarate hydratase by multiplex ligation-dependent probe amplification: detection of exonic deletion in a patient with leiomyomatosis and renal cell cancer. Cancer Genet Cytogenet 2008; 183: 83–88

[59] Pavlovich CP, Schmidt LS. Searching for the hereditary causes of renal-cell carcinoma. Nat Rev Cancer 2004; 4: 381–393

[60] Gupta GN, Peterson J, Thakore KN et al. Oncological outcomes of partial nephrectomy for multifocal renal cell carcinoma greater than 4 Cm. J Urol 2010; 184: 59–63

Chapter 14

CYLD Cutaneous Syndrome: Familial Cylindromatosis, Brooke-Spiegler Syndrome and Multiple Familial Trichoepitherioma

Takahiro Kurimoto, Naoki Oiso, Muneharu Miyake and Akira Kawada

Additional information is available at the end of the chapter

http://dx.doi.org/10.5772/53575

1. Introduction

The concept of *CYLD* cutaneous syndrome was proposed by Rajan *et al.* in 2009 (Rajan *et al.*, 2009). The syndrome represents an uncommon autosomal dominant disease caused by a germline mutation in the cylindromatosis gene (*CYLD*) (Biggs PJ, *et al.* 1995). *CYLD* cutaneous syndrome is characterized by the development of multiple neoplasms originating from the skin appendages (Rajan *et al.*, 2009). It includes three appendageal tumor predisposition syndromes; familial cylindromatosis (FC, MIM 132700), Brooke-Spiegler syndrome (BSS, MIM 605041), and multiple familial trichoepithelioma (MFT, MIM 601606) (Rajan *et al.*, 2009). BSS is characterized by multiple skin appendage tumors such as cylindroma, trichoepithelioma, and spiradenoma. FC is typified by multiple cylindromas and MFT by multiple trichoepitheliomas. Here, we summarize current clinical and genetic recognition in *CYLD* cutaneous syndrome.

2. *CYLD* cutaneous syndrome

A genome search using two FC families identified strong evidence for linkage to the locus on chromosome 16q12-q13 (Biggs *et al.*, 1995). Subsequently, germline mutations in the tumor suppressor *CYLD* gene were identified in individuals having FC (Bignell *et al.* 2000). A combination of genetic linkage analysis and loss of heterozygosity in 15 FC families showed only the linkage to the locus, providing no evidence for genetic heterogeneity (Takahashi *et al.* 2000). The germline mutations were then detected in individuals with BSS (HU *et al.*, 2003; Poblete Gutiérrez *et al.*, 2002) and MFT (Salhi *et al.*, 2004; Zhang *et al.*, 2004; Zheng *et al.*, 2004). Affected family members with the same germline mutation in *CYLD* showed FC, BSS or MFT phenotypes, indicating the absence of genotype-phenotype relationship (Fenske *et al.*, 2000; Rajan *et al.*, 2009; Young *et al.*, 2006). The phenotypic diversity from mild type to severe turban tumor is present in the affected family members with *CYLD* cutaneous syndrome (Biggs *et al.*, 1995; Oiso *et al.*, 2004; Rajan *et al.*, 2009; Young *et al.*, 2006). Bowen *et al.* suggested that FC, BSS, and MTF represent phenotypic variation of a single entity (Bowen *et al.*, 2005). Rajan *et al.* proposed the term, *CYLD* cutaneous syndrome, for unifying three skin appendage-associated disorders (Rajan *et al.*, 2009).

3. The function of CYLD

In 2003, CYLD was shown as a deubiquitinating enzyme that negatively regulates nuclear factor-kappa B (NF-κB) activation (Brummelkamp *et al.*, 2003; Kovalenko *et al.*, 2003; Trompouki *et al.*, 2003; Wilkinson, 2003). NF-κB is involved in controlling inflammation, the immune response, and apoptosis (Pasparakis, 2002). Nowadays, many different cellular functions have been ascribed to CYLD such as proliferation and cell cycle, Ca2+ channel signaling, survival and apoptosis, inflammation, T-cell development and activation, antiviral response, and spermatogenesis (Pasparakis, 2002).

CYLD contains three cytoskeleton-associated protein-glycine-rich (CAP-Gly) domains, two proline-rich motifs, a tumor necrosis factor-alpha (TNF-α) receptor-associated factor 2 (TRAF2) binding site, and ubiquitin-specific proteases (USP) domain responsible for its deubiquitinases (DUB) activity (Harhaj et al., 2011; Pasparakis, 2002). The first two CAP-Gly domains mediate binding to microtubules (Gao *et al.*, 2008; Wickström *et al.*, 2010), and the third CAP-Gly domain regulates NEMO interactions. NEMO (also known as IκB kinase gamma (IKKγ)) is the regulatory subunit of the IκB kinase (IKK) (Yoshida *et al.*, 2011). IKK plays crucial role in activating NF-κB in response to various inflammatory stimuli (Zheng *et al.*, 2011). TRAF2 regulates activation of the c-Jun N-terminal kinase (JNK)/c-Jun and the inhibitor of IKK/ NF-κB signaling cascades in response to TNF-α stimulation (Zhang *et al.*, 2011).

4. Conclusion

CYLD cutaneous syndrome represents familial cylindromatosis, Brooke-Spiegler syndrome, and multiple familial trichoepithelioma. Further studies for elucidating the function of *CYLD* will focus on defining the multifunctional activities including tumor suppression for neoplasms from the skin appendages.

Author details

Takahiro Kurimoto, Naoki Oiso*, Muneharu Miyake and Akira Kawada
Department of Dermatology,
Kinki University Faculty of Medicine,
Osaka-Sayama, Japan

* Corresponding Author

5. References

Biggs PJ, Wooster R, Ford D, *et al.* Familial cylindromatosis (turban tumour syndrome) gene localised to chromosome 16q12-q13: evidence for its role as a tumour suppressor gene. *Nat Genet* 1995; 11(4): 441-3.

Bignell GR, Warren W, Seal S, *et al.* Identification of the familial cylindromatosis tumour-suppressor gene. *Nat Genet* 2000; 25(2): 160-5.

Bowen S, Gill M, Lee DA, *et al.* Mutations in the CYLD gene in Brooke-Spiegler syndrome, familial cylindromatosis, and multiple familial trichoepithelioma: lack of genotype-phenotype correlation. J Invest Dermatol 2005; 124(5): 919-20.

Brummelkamp TR, Nijman SM, Dirac AM, *et al.* Loss of the cylindromatosis tumour suppressor inhibits apoptosis by activating NF-kappaB. Nature 2003; 424(6950): 797-801.

Fenske C, Banerjee P, Holden C, *et al.* Brooke-Spiegler syndrome locus assigned to 16q12-q13. J Invest Dermatol 2000; 114(5): 1057-8.

Gao J, Huo L, Sun X, *et al.* The tumor suppressor CYLD regulates microtubule dynamics and plays a role in cell migration. *J Biol Chem* 2008; 283(14): 8802-9.

Harhaj EW, Dixit VM. Deubiquitinases in the regulation of NF-κB signaling. Cell Res 2011; 21(1): 22-39.

Hu G, Onder M, Gill M, *et al.* A novel missense mutation in CYLD in a family with Brooke-Spiegler syndrome. *J Invest Dermatol* 2003; 121(4): 732-4.

Kovalenko A, Chable-Bessia C, Cantarella G, *et al.* The tumour suppressor CYLD negatively regulates NF-kappaB signalling by deubiquitination. *Nature* 2003; 424(6950): 801-5.

Massoumi R. Ubiquitin chain cleavage: CYLD at work. *Trends Biochem Sci* 2010; 35(7): 392-9.

Oiso N, Mizuno N, Fukai K, *et al.* Mild phenotype of familial cylindromatosis associated with an R758X nonsense mutation in the CYLD tumour suppressor gene. Br *J Dermatol* 2004; 151(5): 1084-6.

Pasparakis M, Courtois G, Hafner M, *et al.* TNF-mediated inflammatory skin disease in mice with epidermis-specific deletion of IKK2. *Nature* 2002; 417(6891): 861-6.

Poblete Gutiérrez P, Eggermann T, Höller D, *et al.* Phenotype diversity in familial cylindromatosis: a frameshift mutation in the tumor suppressor gene CYLD underlies different tumors of skin appendages. *J Invest Dermatol* 2002; 119(2): 527-31.

Rajan N, Langtry JA, Ashworth A, *et al.* Tumor mapping in 2 large multigenerational families with CYLD mutations: implications for disease management and tumor induction. *Arch Dermatol* 2009; 145(11): 1277-84.

Salhi A, Bornholdt D, Oeffner F, *et al.* Multiple familial trichoepithelioma caused by mutations in the cylindromatosis tumor suppressor gene. *Cancer Res* 2004; 64(15): 5113-7.

Takahashi M, Rapley E, Biggs PJ, *et al.* Linkage and LOH studies in 19 cylindromatosis families show no evidence of genetic heterogeneity and refine the CYLD locus on chromosome 16q12-q13. *Hum Genet* 2000; 106(1): 58-65.

Trompouki E, Hatzivassiliou E, Tsichritzis T, *et al.* CYLD is a deubiquitinating enzyme that negatively regulates NF-kappaB activation by TNFR family members. *Nature* 2003; 424(6950): 793-6.

Wickström SA, Masoumi KC, Khochbin S, *et al*. CYLD negatively regulates cell-cycle progression by inactivating HDAC6 and increasing the levels of acetylated tubulin *EMBO J* 2010; 29(1): 131-44.

Wilkinson KD. Signal transduction: aspirin, ubiquitin and cancer. *Nature* 2003; 424(6950): 738-9.

Yoshida M, Oiso N, Kimura M, *et al*. Skin ulcer mimicking pyoderma gangrenosum in a patient with incontinentia pigmenti. *J Dermatol* 2011; 38(10): 1019-21.

Young AL, Kellermayer R, Szigeti R, *et al*. CYLD mutations underlie Brooke-Spiegler, familial cylindromatosis, and multiple familial trichoepithelioma syndromes *Clin Genet* 2006; 70(3): 246-9.

Zhang L, Blackwell K, Altaeva A, *et al*. TRAF2 phosphorylation promotes NF-κB-dependent gene expression and inhibits oxidative stress-induced cell death. *Mol Biol Cell* 2011; 22(1): 128-40.

Zhang XJ, Liang YH, He PP, *et al*. Identification of the cylindromatosis tumor-suppressor gene responsible for multiple familial trichoepithelioma. *J Invest Dermatol* 2004; 122(3): 658-64.

Zheng C, Yin Q, Wu H. Structural studies of NF-κB signaling. *Cell Res* 2011; 21(1): 183-95.

Zheng G, Hu L, Huang W, *et al*. CYLD mutation causes multiple familial trichoepithelioma in three Chinese families. *Hum Mutat* 2004; 23(4): 400.